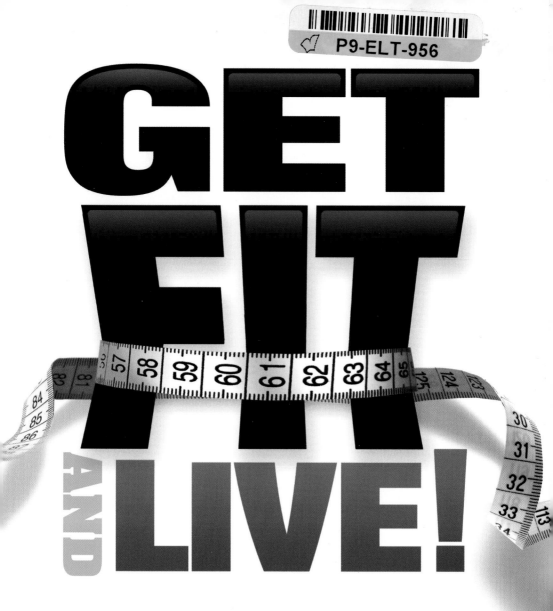

GET FIT AND LIVE!

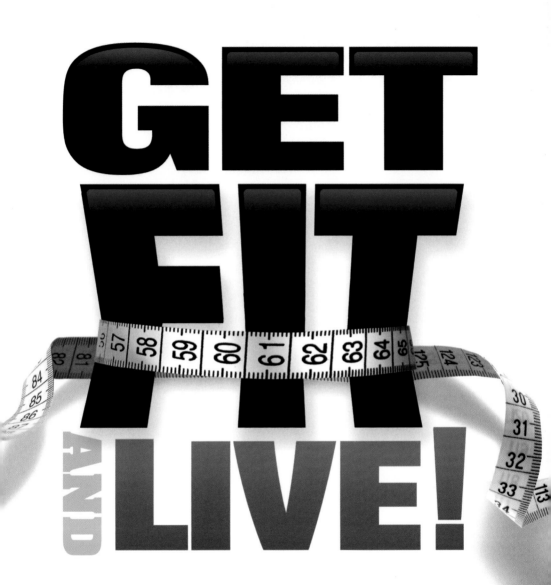

GET FIT AND LIVE!

DON COLBERT, MD & KYLE COLBERT, CPT

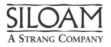

SILOAM
A STRANG COMPANY

Most Strang Communications Book Group products are available at special quantity discounts for bulk purchase for sales promotions, premiums, fund-raising, and educational needs. For details, write Strang Communications Book Group, 600 Rinehart Road, Lake Mary, Florida 32746, or telephone (407) 333-0600.

Get Fit and Live! by Don Colbert, MD, and Kyle Colbert, CPT
Published by Siloam
A Strang Company
600 Rinehart Road
Lake Mary, Florida 32746
www.strangbookgroup.com

Unless otherwise noted, all Scripture quotations are from the New King James Version of the Bible. Copyright © 1979, 1980, 1982 by Thomas Nelson, Inc., publishers. Used by permission.

Scripture quotations marked NASU are from the New American Standard Bible—Updated Edition, Copyright © 1960, 1962, 1963, 1968, 1971, 1972, 1973, 1975, 1977, 1995 by The Lockman Foundation. Used by permission. (www.Lockman.org)

Scripture quotations marked NKJV are from the New King James Version of the Bible. Copyright © 1979, 1980, 1982 by Thomas Nelson, Inc., publishers. Used by permission.

Design Director: Bill Johnson
Cover design by Justin Evans
Interior design by Jeanne Logue and Debbie Marrie
Exercise photos by Kon Studios

Library of Congress Cataloging-in-Publication Data:
An application to register this book for cataloging has been submitted to the Library of Congress.
International Standard Book Number: 978-1-61638-026-7

This book contains the opinions and ideas of its authors. It is solely for informational and educational purposes and should not be regarded as a substitute for professional medical treatment. The nature of your body's health condition is complex and unique. Therefore, you should consult a health professional before you begin any new exercise, nutrition, or supplementation program or if you have questions about your health. Neither the authors

10 11 12 13 14 — 9 8 7 6 5 4 3 2
Printed in the United States of America

DEDICATION

I dedicate this book to my dad, Don Colbert Sr., who went to be with the Lord in August of 2009. He was the greatest witness for Jesus Christ that I have ever seen. I share more about him in the special note in the back of this book.

CONTENTS

INTRODUCTION

From Don Colbert, MD

W HEN I WROTE *The Seven Pillars of Health*, I introduced people to the seven basic pillars of a healthy lifestyle. I believe that by living out the seven principles I shared in that book, anyone can become stronger, healthier, more energetic, younger looking, wiser, smarter, and more disease resistant.

As a medical doctor who is board certified in family practice and anti-aging, I have dedicated my life to helping people become healthy. Because I have spent more than twenty years treating patients, the advice I give in my books is based on my years of experience with real problems and real people.

One area of health that I commonly address when treating my patients is exercise. Why? Because research has shown us over and over again that too many Americans are becoming obese due to poor dietary choices and inactivity!

Next to making the right food choices every day, incorporating regular activity into our daily lives is the most important thing we can do to promote health and healing. Our bodies are designed for movement and resistance in order to stay flexible, strong, and fit.

It is believed that Hippocrates said, "If we could give every individual the right amount of nourishment and exercise, not too little and not too much, we would have found the safest way to health." Even then, he knew that the proper nutrition and exercise are the dynamic duo of good health. For this reason, I felt it made sense to follow on the heels of the release of my book *Eat This and Live!* with the book you now hold in your hands.

In my book *Eat This and Live!* which is based on pillar 3 of *The Seven Pillars of Health*, I showed you how to make simple food choices that leave you looking younger, feeling healthier, and living longer. It didn't take long for people to start asking me for a similar road map to help them navigate through the often-dreaded territory of exercise. As a result I asked my son, Kyle, a certified personal trainer, to join me in creating a simple yet comprehensive workout anyone can follow for better health.

The first several chapters of this book come from pillar 4 of *The Seven Pillars of Health*, where I lay the groundwork to help you obtain a deeper understanding of the benefits and basics of proper exercise. In chapters 8 and 9, Kyle and I have removed the guesswork by giving you a complete workout that you can do in just seven minutes a day. The last several chapters take into consideration various health conditions that you might have and how you should adapt the workout to meet your needs. As a result, this is an extremely practical guidebook that teaches you how to adopt an activity level that is maintainable for years to come. Our goal in writing this book was not to make exercising a chore or to make more work on your part, but to enable you to exchange old habits for new ones.

Our bodies are designed for movement and resistance to keep our muscles and joints flexible and functioning properly into old age. And speaking of old age, many people think that getting old is an excuse to stop exercising. This couldn't be further from the truth! I heard a quote years ago that has stuck with me to this day: "You don't stop exercising because you get old; you get old because you stop exercising."

When Moses was 120 years old, he climbed Mount Nebo from the plains of Moab. Mount Nebo, located in Jordan, is a high mountain—about 800 meters or 2,600 feet at its highest point. I have friends who have tried to climb this mountain, but they just couldn't do it and had to take a helicopter to the top. Yet Moses was able to climb it and see from Mount Nebo into the Promised Land before he died. The Bible tells us:

> Moses was 120 years old when he died, yet his eyesight was clear, and he was as strong as ever.
>
> —DEUTERONOMY 34:7

Moses was 120 years old but had great eyesight and was very strong—so strong he was able to climb a 2,600-foot mountain. God desires for His children to be strong, and we must exercise regularly in order to *be* strong and *stay* strong.

Building an exercise program into your schedule doesn't have to be boring or burdensome; it can be simple, fast, and enjoyable. Be creative and innovative with the information you're about to read, and make it your priority to get fit and live!

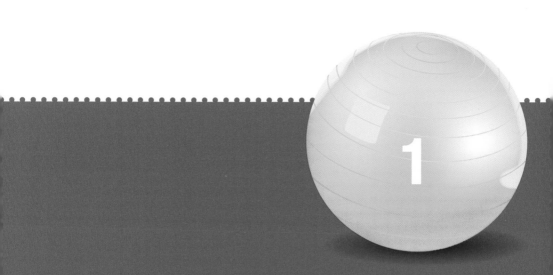

LET'S STIR THE WATERS

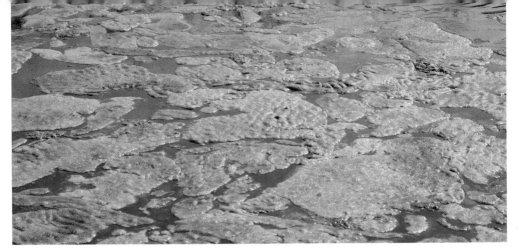

IT'S TIME TO STIR THINGS UP!

AFTER WE SPOKE AT a church in Texas a few years ago, a man in his early thirties came up to us. He must have weighed 450 pounds. He said he had been on bed rest for years because of some kind of infection. Now the infection was gone, but he was having trouble regaining his health. Just by looking at him we could tell he had reached a place of lymphatic stasis—stagnation—so extreme that his legs had blown up to huge proportions. He was so full of toxins that his body was literally bulging with them.

He asked what his problem might be—why he had gained so much weight and why he felt so unhealthy. We told him it was most likely because he hadn't "stirred his waters" with exercise.

We like to refer to exercise as stirring the waters because our bodies are approximately two-thirds water. Think of what happens when water sits for a long time in a cup, puddle, or pond. It eventually gets covered with slime and gunk, breeds disease, and becomes toxic. Think of those green algae-covered ponds you see when you drive through the country. That process is similar to what's going on in many people's bodies.

On the other hand, when water moves, life thrives. Running water is usually fresh water. Rivers and waterfalls are beautiful and inviting—alive. That's a perfect picture of what exercise does. It refreshes your body and clears it of toxins and cellular garbage, sharpening your mind and giving you strength and energy.

Consider again that your body is mostly water. There are many references in the Bible that associate flowing water with life and healing. The Gospel of John tells about the crippled people who waited at the pool of Bethesda because they believed an angel would occasionally stir the waters, healing whomever got into the pool at that moment. To them, the movement of water symbolized life. (See John 5:2–7.)

When water moves, things grow and thrive. On the other hand, dead things are commonly associated with stagnant bodies of water. Exercise is the remedy to prevent death and stir the waters of life in your body. It's time to take your health into your own hands and stir the waters of life with exercise.

How Would Jesus Exercise?

In ancient times, people of the Bible lived in action and motion. They didn't call it exercise, but that's what it was. People did heavy manual labor and usually walked wherever they needed to go.

Jesus did heavy manual labor as a carpenter. From the time He was five until the age of thirty, it's very likely that He walked at least 18,000 miles just on the three annual pilgrimages from Galilee to Jersualem![1] Adding up the total miles Jesus walked during His life would be at least 21,595 miles; the distance around the world at the equator is 24,901.55 miles.[2]

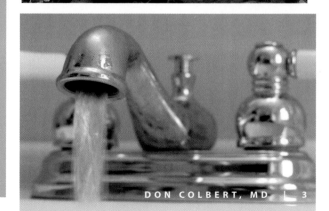

DON COLBERT, MD 3

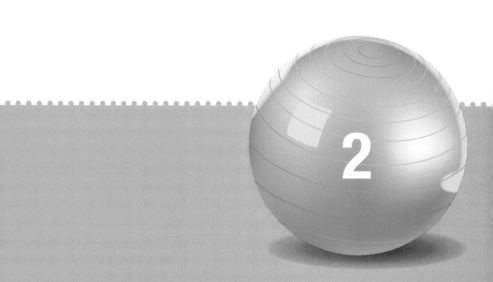

2

THE PERKS OF REGULAR EXERCISE

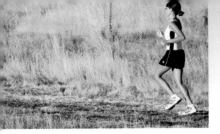

BENEFITS OF EXERCISE

WE USED TO HAVE a sports car that we loved but didn't drive much. After a while we noticed that when we took it out for a spin every few weeks, the engine wouldn't run well. We took it to the shop, and the mechanic inspected it and said, "You haven't been driving this car enough, have you? It was built to run. If you don't drive it, it will break down because you're not using it." We were ruining the car by keeping it parked.

Just like that sports car, your body was designed to move. It needs water, rest, food, and exercise to run smoothly. When you "park" yourself in a chair and don't exercise, eventually you may ruin your engine. Many people these days are sick because they haven't stirred their waters with movement and action. They have become cesspools of disease due to stagnation. Soon they will get to the point where they can't exercise because their bodies are so broken down with heart disease, arthritis, and other degenerative diseases. "Stirring the waters" with exercise has many powerful effects on your health. On the next few pages, we'll tell you about many of them.

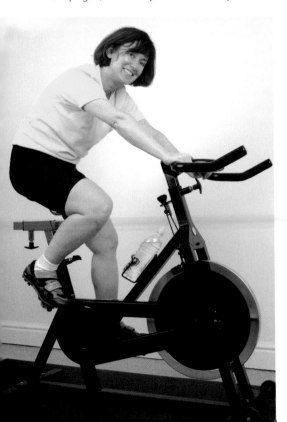

1. Exercise prevents cancer.

Studies show that approximately one-third of cancer deaths can be linked to diet and sedentary lifestyles.[1] Simple movement and exercise decrease the risk of certain cancers such as breast, colon, and possibly endometrial and prostate cancers.[2] In 2005, the National Cancer Institute reported that "physical activity at work or during leisure time is linked to a 50 percent lower risk of getting colon cancer."[3] A study published in the *Journal of the American Medical Association* found that women who engaged in the equivalent of brisk walking for about one to two hours per week decreased their risk of breast cancer by 18 percent compared with inactive women.[4] (See chapter 16 for more information about cancer.)

2. Exercise prevents heart attacks and heart disease.

Cardiovascular disease is the most common cause of death in the United States today.[5] Exercise protects you against it. All kinds of studies show that moderate regular exercise is perhaps the single most important deterrent of heart-related problems.

3. Exercise improves lymphatic flow.

The lymphatic system is a major microbe crime fighter and cellular garbage collector in the body. It removes toxins and cellular waste, and it "keeps the peace" by rounding up bacteria, viruses, and other bad guys, bringing them to the lymph nodes where they are killed by white blood cells. Lymphatic fluid is so important that your body contains about three times more lymph than blood. The lymphatic fluid moves around via very small vessels, which usually run alongside small veins and arteries.

But the lymphatic system has a challenge: it is circulated by muscle contractions, not by your heartbeat. When you don't move, the lymphatic system becomes sluggish. But aerobic exercise can triple the rate of lymphatic flow. That means that the lymphatic system—your in-house police force and cellular garbage collector—does a much better job protecting your body from attack and removing cellular trash.

GET FIT AND LIVE!

Dr. Colbert Approved

A "Natural" Heart Bypass

If you have coronary artery disease, regular exercise will encourage your body to create collateral arteries, which may form a natural bypass around clogged arteries. Years ago I had a patient with an 80 to 90 percent blockage in his right coronary artery. After being on a regular aerobic exercise program for over one year, he actually formed a natural bypass around that plugged artery. That's what exercise can do!

Benefits of Exercise (Continued)

4. Exercise helps you cope with stress.

Regular exercise enhances neurotransmitter production and helps to lower cortisol levels, which helps you feel less stressed. One researcher conducted an experiment with laboratory rats. He took some rats, shocked them with electrodes, shone bright lights, and played loud noises to them around the clock. At the end of one month, all the rats were dead from the stress. He then took another group of rats and made them exercise on a treadmill. After they were well exercised, he subjected them to a month of the same shocks, noises, and lights. These rats didn't die—they ran around well and healthy.[6] If life is stressing you out, it's time to add exercise to your day. Exercise literally burns off those stress chemicals.

5. Exercise promotes weight loss and decreases appetite.

Weight training and calisthenics are exercises that increase your muscle mass, which raises your metabolic rate and enables you to burn more fat. It is perhaps the safest method of raising your metabolic rate, which is the rate at which your body converts food into energy. Realize that the basal metabolic rate decreases by approximately 5 percent for every decade of life after the age of twenty. People who are sedentary have a significant loss of muscle mass as they age. In these sedentary individuals there is about a seven-pound loss of muscle mass every ten years past the age of twenty. So by age sixty, most have lost about twenty-eight pounds of muscle and replaced it with much more fat.

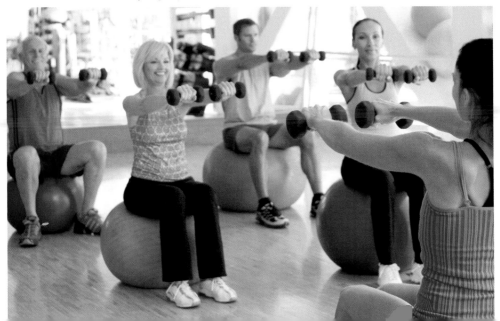

Aerobic exercise such as brisk walking and cycling is also a very effective way to lose weight and keep it off.

Moderate aerobic exercise is also quite effective at decreasing your appetite, but you must be in your target heart rate. Individuals who exercise outside of their target heart rate by exercising too intensely may develop a ravenous appetite an hour or so after exercising due to hypoglycemia, or low blood sugar. (See chapter 11 for more information.)

6. Exercise may help prevent diabetes and help control blood sugar in diabetics.

Exercise holds special benefits for diabetics. By helping muscles to take up glucose from the bloodstream and use it for energy, exercise prevents sugar from accumulating in the blood. By burning calories, exercise helps control weight, which is also an important factor in the management of type 2 diabetes. Exercise is also very important for individuals with type 1 diabetes; it helps to lower insulin requirements. Exercise improves the body's ability to use insulin. (See chapter 12 for more information.)

7. Exercise increases perspiration.

Sweating is one of the body's ways of getting rid of waste products. The skin has been called "the third kidney" because it releases so many toxins from the body. At normal activity levels, people lose two to three cups of water a day in perspiration. But during an hour of vigorous exercise, people sweat out approximately a quart of water.[7]

GET FIT AND LIVE!

Wow! Moderate Exercise, Major Benefits

A study by Joslin Diabetes Center researchers showed that obese adults who lost just 7 percent of their weight and did moderate-intensity physical exercise for six months improved their major blood vessel function by approximately 80 percent, regardless of whether or not they had type 2 diabetes.[8]

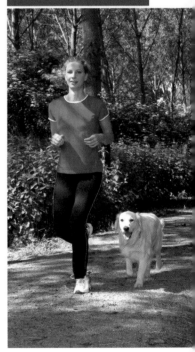

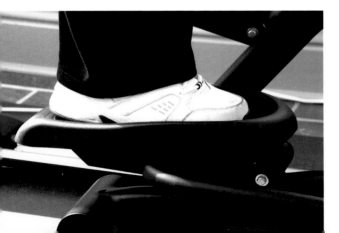

BENEFITS OF EXERCISE (CONTINUED)

8. Exercise slows the aging process.

In a study published in the *American Journal of Physiology*, Christiaan Leeuwenburgh, a professor at the University of Florida College of Health and Human Performance, found that antioxidant intervention, which can come from taking antioxidant supplements or from a steady routine of exercise, slows parts of the aging process. "We were surprised to see that regular exercise training was about as effective in reducing levels of oxidation as a diet of antioxidants," Leeuwenburgh said.[9]

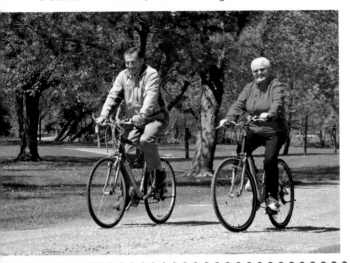

Everyone wants to look young and fit forever. But did you know the reality is that adults typically lose approximately ½ to 1 pound of muscle tissue every year past the age of twenty-five? Stated another way, our bodies naturally progress toward more fat and less muscle. That isn't the greatest news for those who are already struggling with bodies overloaded with fat. But it can be a driving force for turning your body from flab to fit.

Understand that the more muscle mass you have, generally the higher your metabolic rate and the more calories you will burn at rest. For each pound of muscle mass that you either gain or do not lose, you will burn approximately 30 to 50 calories a day.

If you are inactive most of the time, your muscles are slowly melting away. Your metabolic rate is decreasing, while your muscle tissue is (typically) being replaced with fat. Many people do not notice this because the size of their arm or leg remains the same, when in fact it is simply a case of fat replacing muscle tissue.

This is particularly true for women. A woman's metabolism typically begins to decrease at the age of twenty at a rate of about 5 percent per decade of life. To understand this more, let's use the example of an average fifty-year-old female—we'll call her Sarah. Since her late twenties, Sarah's weight has gone from around 120 to her current weight of 150 pounds. During those years, she gained 30 pounds of fat, but she also lost around 15 to 30 pounds of muscle. That may sound like it averages out except when you consider the corresponding drop in metabolic rate. When she was twenty, Sarah could eat 2,000 calories a day and maintain her 120-pound frame. At the age of fifty, however, if she eats 2,000 calories a day, she will most likely gain weight because of the muscle tissue she has lost. Remember, for each pound of muscle tissue lost, your metabolic rate decreases by 30 to 50 calories per day. So in addition to losing 15 pounds of muscle, Sarah also lost the ability for her metabolic rate to burn about 450 to 750 more calories a day.

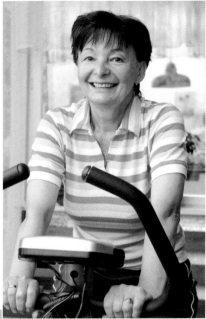

Now you can see why maintaining or gaining muscle mass is so crucial. Muscle does not just look better than fat; it is also essential for maintaining a healthy body. And the only way to keep muscle intact is to use it and keep it strengthened on a regular basis, which means increasing your activity level or exercising. When you decide to do the opposite and remain inactive, you put yourself in a body cast, so to speak, as your metabolic rate nosedives and you become a fat magnet.

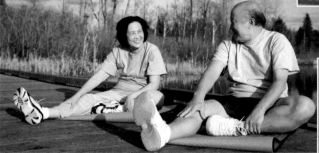

Exercise Slows Alzheimer's and May Help Prevent Parkinson's

Carl Cotman, a neuroscientist at the University of California, has conducted research with laboratory mice that suggests physical exercise can slow the progression of Alzheimer's disease. Testing has also shown that exercise may prevent Parkinson's symptoms from developing in animals predisposed with that disease.[10]

Exercise Improves Memory Retention

Prolonged exposure of your neurons (nerve cells) to high levels of stress hormones, like cortisol, decreases your brain's ability to take up glucose, and neurons begin to atrophy and eventually die. This results in a decrease in memory retention. Regular aerobic exercise helps to lower cortisol levels, which may help to improve memory.

BENEFITS OF EXERCISE (CONTINUED)

9. Exercise builds strong bones.

Bone density screening has gone high-tech, and as a result, more and more researchers can now measure the effects of various factors in the bone-building process and prevention of osteoporosis. Their research shows that exercise works better than calcium in building strong bones. "Although calcium intake is often cited as the most important factor for healthy bones, our study suggests that exercise is really the predominant lifestyle determinant of bone strength in young women," said Tom Lloyd, PhD, an epidemiologist with the Penn State University College of Medicine, whose findings were reported in the *Journal of Pediatrics*.[11] (See chapter 13 for more information.)

10. Exercise improves your digestion and promotes regular bowel movements.

Exercise helps prevent constipation.[12] Studies have shown that physical activity may help to ease digestion problems and problems with the GI tract. That's the conclusion of a study in an October 2005 issue of *Clinical Gastroenterology and Hepatology*. The study of 1,801 men and women found that obese people who got some form of physical activity were less likely to suffer GI problems than inactive obese people. "It is well documented that maintaining a healthy diet and regular physical activity can benefit GI health," study author Rona L. Levy, a professor at the University of Washington in Seattle, said.[13]

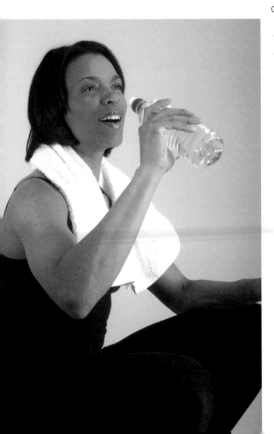

11. Exercise gives you restful sleep.

One of the best ways to improve the quality of your sleep is to exercise. Researchers found that women who participated in forty-five minutes of aerobics in the morning were about 70 percent less likely to have trouble sleeping than those who exercised less.[14] You shouldn't exercise within three hours of bedtime because it can cause insomnia; however, stretching and relaxing your muscles at any time of the day help to ease stiffness and have also been shown to make people 30 percent less likely to have trouble sleeping.[15] For more information on sleep, see the book *The New Bible Cure for Sleep Disorders*.

12. Exercise helps prevent colds and flu.

Research shows that aerobic exercise such as brisk walking, jogging, or cycling boosts the body's defenses against viruses and bacteria during the cold and flu season. Too much exercise can increase your risk of infection, but moderate amounts (thirty minutes, three to four times per week) produce positive results by increasing the circulation of immune cells from bone marrow, the lungs, and the spleen.[16]

13. Exercise reduces depression.

Exercise increases serotonin and dopamine levels, which helps to relieve symptoms of anxiety and depression. One study looked at aerobic exercise as a means of treating clinical depression. An aerobic exercise program was compared to standard medication in a group of older adult patients. Medication relieved symptoms of depression more rapidly at the outset, but aerobic exercise was shown to be equally effective to medication over the course of the four-month study. Since some medications for depression have adverse effects or cease to be as effective with prolonged use, this was an important finding— aerobic exercise may be a very viable long-term therapy.[17]

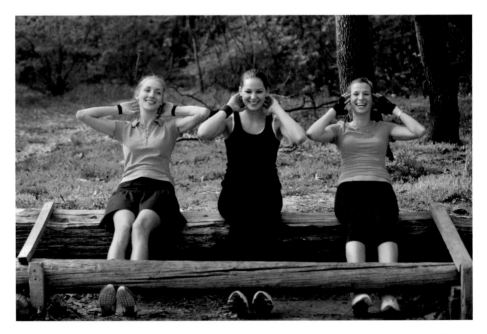

Benefits of Exercise (Continued)

14. Exercise increases lung capacity.

As we age, our lung capacity diminishes. Cardiovascular activity and exercise can combat this because aerobic exercise increases lung capacity. So while our lung capacity may continue to diminish, it does so at a slower pace.[18]

15. Exercise alleviates pain.

It might sound crazy to suggest exercising when you are in pain, but regular exercise is a bigger pain-fighting weapon than you might think. Aerobic exercise causes the release of endorphins, which are morphinelike molecules produced by the body. In an article published by the Mayo Clinic, it was reported that regular exercise actually reduces chronic pain for many people. The article quotes Dr. Edward Laskowski of Mayo Clinic as saying, "Years ago, people who were in pain were told to rest, but now we know the exact opposite is true. When you rest, you become deconditioned—which may actually contribute to chronic pain."[19] (For information on pain from fibromyalgia or arthritis, refer to chapters 14 and 17.)

16. Exercise increases your energy level.

Aerobic exercise in your target heart rate range will actually increase your energy. Most people have the excuse that they are simply too tired to exercise; they don't realize that regular aerobic exercise can dramatically increase their energy.[20]

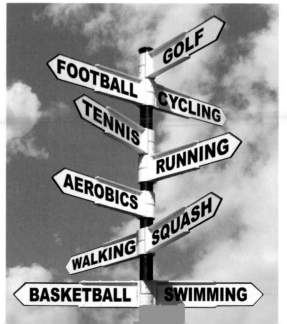

Let's Recap: The Perks of Regular Exercise

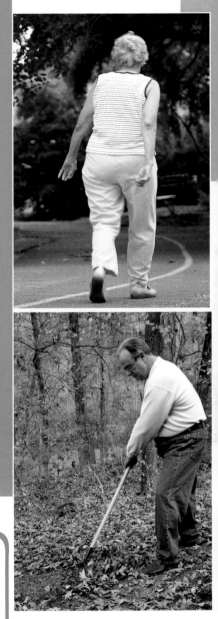

In case you needed a reminder, here are just a few of the tremendous benefits that come with regular exercise:

- It decreases the risk of heart disease and stroke, as well as the development of hypertension.

- It helps prevent type 2 diabetes.

- It helps protect you from developing certain types of cancer.

- It helps prevent osteoporosis and aids in maintaining healthy bones.

- It helps prevent arthritis and aids in maintaining healthy joints.

- It slows down the overall aging process.

- It improves your mood and reduces the symptoms of anxiety and depression.

- It increases energy and mental alertness.

- It improves your digestion.

- It gives you restful sleep.

- It helps prevent colds and flu.

- It alleviates pain.

And the health benefit you likely already knew about…

- It promotes weight loss and decreases appetite!

GET FIT and LIVE!

Did You Know…?

If you have been watching what you eat and working out, and yet the scale isn't moving, don't be discouraged. Muscle weighs more than fat, and it increases the metabolic rate, helping to burn fat too. So, generally speaking, the more muscle you build, the more body fat you will lose.

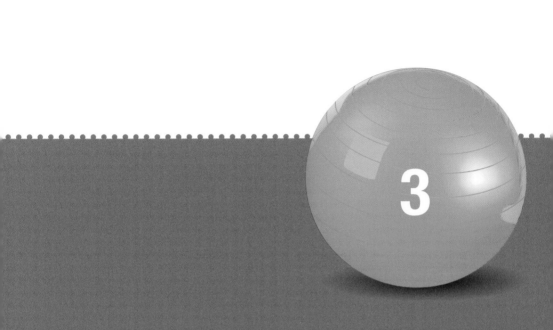

3

BEFORE YOU BEGIN

SAFETY FIRST

IS IT OK TO exercise when I'm sick? Are some exercises dangerous when dealing with certain physical conditions or taking certain medications? These questions, and others like them, are very important for you to discuss with your personal health care provider. The information in this book is provided to increase your knowledge and arm you with the tools you need to help improve your physical fitness, but it can never take the place of the advice of a physician who is familiar with your specific health needs.

We cannot think of a single physical condition you might be experiencing that would not benefit from some level of activity. However, even though physical exercise is beneficial for everyone and is completely safe for most people, there are times when you should check with a doctor before beginning a new exercise routine.

So how do you know when a trip to the doctor's office should be the first step in your new workout routine? The American College of Sports Medicine (ACSM) recommends checking with your doctor if two or more of the following apply to you:

- You are a man older than 45 or a woman older than 55.
- You have a family history of heart disease before age 55.
- You have high blood pressure.
- You have high cholesterol.
- You are currently smoking or have quit within the past six months.
- You are overweight or obese.

In addition to the ACSM's list, we also recommend checking with your doctor if:

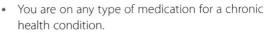

- You are on any type of medication for a chronic health condition.
- You have a disability that will require you to modify the chosen activity.
- You've had a heart attack.
- You're pregnant.
- You suffer from arthritis, osteoporosis, diabetes, or any of the other health conditions we specifically address in later chapters of this book.
- You aren't aware of any existing health issues, but during a workout, you experience chest pain, dizziness, loss of balance, or persistent joint or muscle pain.

Planning a Safe Fitness Routine[1]

GET FIT AND LIVE!

According to the U. S. Department of Health and Human Services, to stay safe and reduce the risk of injury and other adverse events during physical exercise, you should:

- Choose exercises that are appropriate for your current fitness level and goals.
- Increase your workout gradually over time to meet your fitness goals. If you have been inactive up to this point, you should "start low and go slow" by gradually increasing how often you work out, how long you work out, and how intense you work out.
- Use protective gear and sports equipment properly. Personal protective gear (helmets, goggles, shin guards, elbow and knee pads, mouth guards, etc.) should fit properly, be well maintained, and be worn correctly.
- Make sensible choices about when, where, and how to be active. Choose safe locations for outdoor activities, and follow the rules and policies of any fitness facility or sports organization you join.

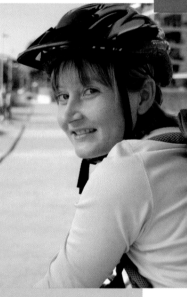

We would also add that you should make sure you have provided your body with the proper fuel mixture (food and nutritional supplements), that you are properly hydrated before, during, and after your workout, and that you take time to properly warm up and cool down. We will discuss these topics more fully in just a few pages.

When the Weather Outside Is Frightful...

Weather conditions, such as extreme heat or cold, can affect the safety of outdoor activities. Of course, you can always switch to indoor activities, but if you really prefer to be out of doors, try making a few simple adjustments in your routine.

For example, if the weather is hot and humid, in addition to protecting yourself from the sun's harmful UV rays, here are a few tips for reducing your chances of dehydration, heat exhaustion, or heatstroke.

- Try a different time of day. Work out in the early morning or evening rather than in the midday heat.
- Avoid full sun. Choose a shadier court or trail, and use appropriate sunscreen and head and eye coverings.
- Stop more frequently for rest and replenishing your fluids.
- Go for a lower intensity in your activity. (Walk instead of running.)
- Opt for a completely different type of activity. (Swim instead of running.)

How Fit Are You? It's Time to Measure Up

TO HELP PEOPLE ESTABLISH their fitness goals, it's important to first determine their current level of fitness. We weigh them on the scale and then measure their waist, body mass index (BMI), and body fat percentage. The BMI, body fat, and number of pounds on the scale are all secondary to what matters most: the waist measurement.

I have discovered that weighing a person weekly is probably one of the worst motivators for getting fit. Oh sure, the first few weeks of working out can seem almost miraculous for some individuals as they watch the pounds fall off. The problem, however, is that many people are in fact losing muscle or water weight, which is guaranteed to lower your metabolic rate and eventually sabotage your fitness goals. When these people hit a plateau a few weeks or months later, they wind up discouraged and often quit the program entirely—all because they are rating their efforts and results based on a weekly scale reading.

This is why after taking the initial measurements I'm discussing here, we have people set a fitness goal that is focused on reducing their need for pain medications, increasing stamina, eliminating chronic health conditions, or losing inches from their waist (rather than pounds). We advise you to take the same approach in establishing your own fitness goals.

1. Measure your waist at the navel

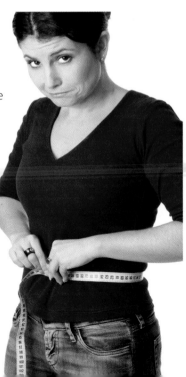

Measure your waistline at your navel, or belly button. If you are a man and your waist measurement is greater than or equal to 40 inches, you are at a much greater risk of heart disease, hypertension, type 2 diabetes, metabolic syndrome, and many other diseases. If you are a woman and your waist measurement is greater than or equal to 35 inches, you're prone to the same risks. In fact, after years of linking only weight and BMI to higher mortality rates and serious illnesses, scientists are ning to understand—once again—that abdominal fat is a contributor to the onset of these diseases.

Let us also remind you of something: your waist at your navel (your belly button), not your lower or hips. We have worked with many people who the two and shot themselves in the foot because took helpful, accurate measurements. A man can have a around the navel but still wear a 34-inch-waist pant simply keeps his pants fastened below his bulging belly. (Come on, what I'm talking about.) The popularity of low-cut jeans recent years really has some people confused about the waistline!

Yes, it's that simple. You really do not need a scale, a percent body fat machine, or any other fancy tools—just a simple tape measure.

2. Calculate your BMI

Refer to Appendix B or go online and find many Web sites that have helpful tools and charts to help you calculate your BMI. Several of our books also contain information on calculating your BMI, such as *The Seven Pillars of Health* and *Dr.*

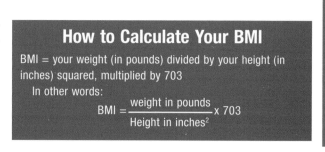

How to Calculate Your BMI

BMI = your weight (in pounds) divided by your height (in inches) squared, multiplied by 703
   In other words:

$$BMI = \frac{weight\ in\ pounds}{Height\ in\ inches^2} \times 703$$

Colbert's "I Can Do This" Diet. But if you want to do the math yourself, it's not that difficult. Simply refer to the formula in the sidebar on this page.

3. Measure your body fat percentage (optional)

You can measure your body fat percentage using a bioimpedance analysis, underwater weighing, or skinfold calipers. Most health clubs have the equipment needed to do so.

4. Measure your flexibility (optional)

After warming up, get a ruler and remove your shoes and sit on a flat surface, with your legs extended in front of your body, toes pointing up and feet slightly apart. Place the ruler on the floor between your legs, with the ruler extending beyond your feet. Then place one hand on top of the other and reach forward slowly. At the point of your farthest reach, hold for a couple of seconds and then measure how far you reached. Note your measurement—how many inches your were able to reach beyond your toes or how many inches short you were of reaching your toes.

5. Record your pulse before and after a brisk one-mile walk (optional)

See the sidebar below for instructions on taking your pulse.

How to Take Your Pulse

Place two fingers on the carotid artery in your neck or on the radial artery in your wrist. Once you find your pulse, count number of beats in ten seconds and multiply by six to get your heart rate per minute.

SET YOUR FITNESS GOALS

WHEN YOU ARE ABOUT to embark on a lifestyle change, it's crucial to establish significant goals. After all, you want your results to be significant, don't you? We have seen countless people dive head-first into a new exercise program with no set goals in mind. We have seen just as many people launch into a workout routine with unrealistic goals. Both usually end up as failures. Success requires vision, and when it comes to getting fit, that vision must also incorporate reality.

An unrealistic goal for your fitness program sets you up for discouragement. People who become discouraged will usually stop the program altogether and eventually revert back to their previous lack of fitness. If you are a five-foot-two-inch female weighing 300 pounds, for instance, understand that you will not be a size 2 or 4 in a year—maybe never. Realistically, look to be a size 10 or 12 with a waist measurement of 35 inches instead of 45 inches. That is an attainable goal. And when you reach that goal, then you can set another.

Likewise, if you hate going to the gym but have set a goal to work out five days a week for an hour each time, you have just created an unrealistic goal and have paved the way for discouragement and failure. Instead, set a goal of ten thousand steps a day on a pedometer, which simply means more movement or more walking.

Also, avoid making promises that can be easily broken. For instance, do not tell yourself that now that you've started working out you will never have another piece of cake, pie, cookie, or whatever food weakness you have. Whenever you say that, you have just set your autopilot on desiring that food and will most likely want that food even more. Instead, as you learn how to develop good eating and exercise habits, avoid using the word *never.*

None of this means that you have to settle for a lowered expectation. You can and will feel better than you ever have. But the important thing is to first set a goal and then keep it in perspective—both of which can come through taking the initial measurements we discussed on the previous page.

It all starts with the waist

Remember all of the health conditions we mentioned that are now being linked to an expanding waistline? They are just some of many reasons why your first goal should be to decrease this area of your body that is holding all this toxic fat and keeping you susceptible to disease. Your first goal, if you are a man, is to get your waist measurement to less than 40 inches and eventually to 37.5 or less. If you are a woman, your first goal is to get your waist measurement to less than 35 inches and eventually to 32.5 inches or less.

Now that you have your waist measurement goal and have recorded your other measurements, you don't have to think about these numbers. Your focus should be simply on taking one day at a time. Too many people pay so much attention to the final result that they forget to focus on what they are doing day by day. As a result, they battle discouragement.

If you get nothing else from this chapter, understand this: Reaching your fitness goals takes time. Not only that, but everyone is different and notices the benefits of exercise at different rates. For instance, men usually lose weight much faster on an exercise program than women do, since men typically have more muscle and a higher metabolic rate. You should be gaining muscle in the process of getting fit, which is another reason to forgo the scale, because muscle weighs more than fat.

You may not be able to control how fast you will reach your goal, but you can control how you follow the path to your goals day to day. When you focus on implementing these fitness and lifestyle choices each day, they will eventually become habits. Many experts say that it takes twenty-one days to form a habit. Others agree upon forty, while still others say it takes ninety days to make that habit a natural part of your lifestyle. However long it takes, the point is that when you simply focus on getting fit for today—without worrying about how you'll face tomorrow or next week—then after a while, after doing this over time, it becomes part of your daily life. And when that begins to happen, you will find your mind's autopilot set on getting fit for life.

Many people get so focused on the goal that they forget the process and, as a result, constantly fight discouragement. By focusing on one day at a time, you consistently make the right choices every day. Obviously, there will be some times when you miss an opportunity to exercise. But do not get discouraged; simply realize that you are just one workout away from getting back on the program and again choosing to make the right choices for your fitness goals.

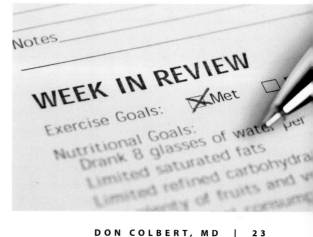

THE RIGHT NUTRITIONAL FUEL FOR YOUR WORKOUT

REMEMBER THE SPORTS CAR that needed to be driven regularly to keep it in optimal condition? Equally important to its performance was keeping it filled up with the right fuel. In the same way, your body needs the right kind of nutritional "fuel." What's the right kind of fuel? We recommend a combination of carbohydrates, proteins, and fats.

- **Carbohydrates** (found in pasta, bread, cereal, rice, potatoes, etc.) often get a bad rap, especially if you've tried many of the recent low-carb fad diets. But it's important to include a proper amount of carbs in your diet when you're starting a fitness program, because they supply the glucose your body needs for energy, especially for activities that use short bursts of high energy. During physical activity, if you don't have enough glycogen (a derivative of glucose), you can become tired very quickly.

- **Protein** (found in meat, omega-3 eggs, dairy, beans, etc.) can be used for energy as well, but more importantly as it pertains to exercise, your body uses protein to build and repair your muscles.

- **Fats** (healthy fats are found in olive oil, cold-pressed vegetable oil, fish, flaxseed, etc.) are an important source of energy, especially for longer activities that require endurance.

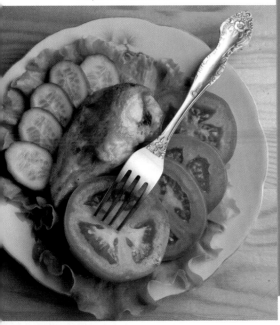

Supplementing Your Fitness Routine With Vitamins and Minerals

Vitamins and minerals don't give you energy, but they affect your ability to exercise by building strong bones (vitamin D and calcium), helping your blood distribute oxygen to the rest of your body (iron), and regulating the water levels in your body and muscles (potassium, calcium, and sodium).

Studies show that the majority of Americans don't get the recommended amounts of most vitamins and minerals. To make sure you are getting enough vitamins and minerals, we recommend eating a well-balanced diet from a variety of foods and supporting this diet with a daily dose of a good-quality multivitamin.

When You Eat Is as Important as *What* You Eat

With many things in life, timing is everything, and scheduling your meals and exercise is no exception. These tips will help you avoid low blood sugar, cramping, and muscle soreness, while keeping energy levels high for a successful workout.

- We recommend eating a full-size meal that combines a 40:30:30 ratio of carbs, proteins, and healthy fats if you eat about three hours before you exercise. Smaller "minimeals" (healthy snacks that use the same ratio of carbs, protein, and fats) are better if you only have two hours or less before your workout. If you work out first thing in the morning and only have time to eat breakfast right before your workout, a good choice is an easily digested protein shake with a banana added to it. This is a slightly higher amount of carbs than we normally recommend. The extra carbs balanced by protein and fat will boost your energy level during your workout and prevent you from burning your muscle tissues as fuel.

- We never recommend going more than three and a half hours without eating either a meal or snack. Skipping meals and healthy snacks can deplete your body of energy and cause you to tire too easily during your workout, making it more likely that you will be tempted to give up. Skipping meals can also cause low blood sugar, which causes you to crave unhealthy foods, which will only add pounds and counteract the health benefits of exercising in the first place.

- Avoid high-fiber foods in your last meal before you exercise because they can cause excess gas, which might give you stomach pains during a workout. Fiber has many health benefits, and most Americans don't get enough fiber, so be sure to eat high-fiber foods for your other meals throughout the day.

- If you have muscle cramps during workouts, a potassium or magnesium deficiency is most likely the cause. Eat a banana, an orange, or a handful of nuts before your workout to help eliminate cramping.

- Avoid high-sugar foods and beverages such soda and energy drinks. Sugary foods will give you a quick energy boost, but you'll quickly experience the familiar "crash" in energy when your blood sugar levels plummet.

- We don't recommend most energy bars because they are loaded with sugar and other unhealthy ingredients. If you want to snack on a protein bar before your workout, we recommend the Divine Health Snack Bar. (See appendix C.)

- After exercising, we recommend eating a meal with a 40:30:30 ratio of carbs, protein, and fats within the first two hours. This combination will help keep your blood sugar from dropping too low while helping to repair and build muscle tissue.

Drinking Adequately for Your Workout

IT PRACTICALLY GOES WITHOUT saying that proper hydration during exercise is a must. There are many benefits of keeping your body adequately hydrated. For regular daily water consumption, as a general rule of thumb it's recommended that you divide your weight (in pounds) in half, and drink that many ounces of water each day. Specific recommendations for how much, how often, and what kind of water I recommend in much greater detail in the books *The Seven Pillars of Health* and *Eat This and Live!* Below are our specific recommendations for water consumption before, during, and after your fitness routine.

- Assuming you avoid being dehydrated on a daily basis because you follow the rule of thumb mentioned above, we advise drinking 15 to 20 ounces of pure, filtered water two to three hours before you exercise and another 8 to 10 ounces fifteen minutes before you exercise.

- During exercise, your body's need for water depends on how intensely you work out and how long you work out, among other things. If you are going to be exercising for less than one hour at moderate intensity, then it is recommended that you drink 8 to 10 ounces of water during your workout at ten- to fifteen-minute intervals.

- If you sweat a lot or exercise at high altitudes, you are at a higher risk of dehydration and should increase your intake of water.

- If you work out in hotter temperatures, you will need to increase the amount of water you drink during your workout to avoid dehydration.

- We always recommend avoiding sodas and energy drinks, but this is especially important regarding exercise because any caffeinated beverage (including coffee or tea) can contribute to dehydration.

- After exercise, drink 16 ounces of water within two hours and resume regular drinking patterns.

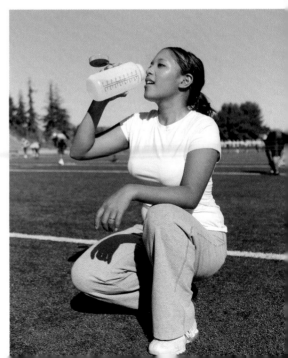

What About Sports Drinks?

Sports drinks such as Gatorade and Powerade can help replenish carbs and electrolytes if you are exercising at a high intensity for sixty minutes or more. However, it's really not necessary to replace sodium, potassium, and other electrolytes during shorter, less intense workouts since it's unlikely that you'll deplete your body's reserves of these minerals. That's why we don't recommend sports drinks if you are only working out for twenty to thirty minutes a day, which is the amount of exercise recommended for the average adult. Water is still the best choice for staying hydrated.

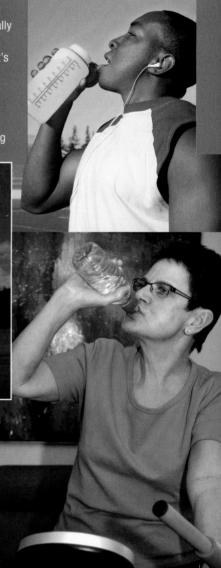

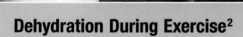

Dehydration During Exercise[2]

Studies link a drop in blood volume to losing 2 or more percent of your body weight due to sweating. When your blood volume drops, the heart has to work harder to pump enough blood to your body, and it can also cause muscle cramps, dizziness, fatigue, heat exhaustion, and heat stroke. If you are concerned because of excessive sweating during workouts, weigh yourself before and after a workout to see how much fluid you lose through sweating. Then replenish your body by drinking 20 to 24 ounces of water for every pound you've lost.

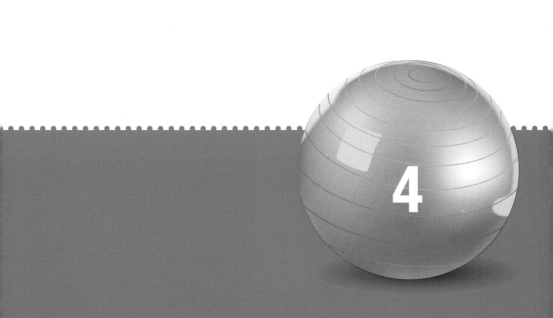

HOW MUCH EXERCISE DO YOU NEED?

THREE KEY FACTORS OF YOUR WORKOUT

ONE OF THE BIGGEST and most common exercise mistakes among people who embark upon a new fitness routine is the tendency to get on a treadmill and run as hard as they can for as long as possible. Their intent is to get the most out of their workout by doing this, but in the long run (pardon the pun), they won't. Sprinting, running, or jogging at a high intensity for long periods of time so that you are short of breath can actually do more harm than good. For those used to being inactive who are just beginning an exercise routine, it's also the quickest way to surefire burnout. To keep this from happening, always have the following three points in mind to ensure that your workout is helping you to meet your fitness goals.

1. Frequency (how often to exercise)

Frequency plays a big role in the effectiveness of your workouts. Working out too often can cause muscles to break down; working out too seldom can make your workout virtually ineffective.

To reduce muscle soreness and give your muscles the time they need to recover and build up after a workout, we recommend exercising in intervals of every other day. If you want to exercise every day, then we suggest you work out different muscle groups each day (alternating between upper body one day and lower body the next day). Your muscles typically need forty-eight hours between workouts to repair themselves or they can start to break down.

2. Duration (how long to exercise)

Duration is the amount of time you spend working out. Experts recommend at least thirty minutes of continuous activity several days a week. We recommend that you start slowly with twenty to thirty minutes and progress as your fitness level increases. You can even break these twenty-minute workouts into two ten-minute chunks per day if that makes things more manageable for you.

3. Intensity (how hard to exercise)

Intensity is simply how hard you are exercising. It probably goes without saying that different activities require different levels of intensity, but you should also remember that even if you do the same exercise repeatedly, you can change the intensity by adjusting the speed or resistance level of the activity. We always recommend that you start with low intensity and go slow. This helps prevent injury and soreness.

Start Slow

It's important not to start off at too great an intensity, because this can lead to injury and excessive soreness and cause you to burn out quickly, as mentioned earlier. We recommend that you start slow—really slow. Exercise just a few minutes a day for a few weeks. Let your body get accustomed to what you're doing. You need to gradually condition unused muscle groups. Weekend warriors injure themselves by going from no exercise to intense exercise. Not only are they more prone to sprains, strains, tendonitis, and bursitis, but also the intense exercise can trigger a heart attack or stroke. You must ease into it.

Over time, you will be able to increase the frequency, duration, and intensity of your exercise as needed to achieve your fitness goals. Also, keep in mind that our recommendations are general guidelines. If you have any chronic health conditions at all, be sure to follow the advice of your health care provider when it comes to setting the frequency, duration, and intensity of your fitness program.

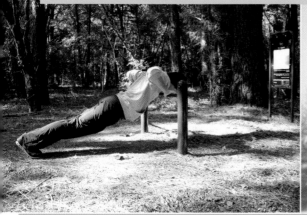

Change It Up

In the same way that eating a wide variety of food helps ensure that you are getting the healthiest diet possible, participating in a wide variety of activities is the best path to fitness. Your body will adapt to any activity that becomes routine, which means that doing the same exercises in the same way for a long period of time will make those exercises less effective in building strength and fitness. To avoid this, we recommend that you change things up every few weeks, alternating among the different forms of aerobic exercise we're going to explain in the next chapter.

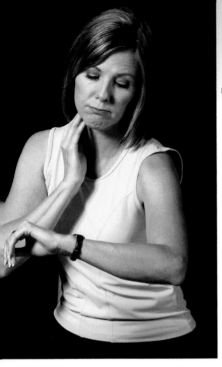

AIM FOR YOUR TARGET HEART RATE

THE GOAL OF THIS chapter is to help you answer the question, How much do I need to exercise? Unfortunately, this cannot be answered with a single universal number. On the previous pages we covered three key factors involved with exercise: frequency, duration, and intensity. On this page, we want to help you calculate your target heart rate. Knowing your target heart rate will help you adjust your workout so that you are exercising at your ideal intensity level.

Every exercise either requires or can be performed at a different level of intensity. Given that, it makes sense, then, that every person hoping to get fit by exercising has an ideal intensity at which they should exercise. This is called your target heart rate zone. Take a look at the box on the next page that gives you the formula for calculating your individual target heart rate.

When beginning an exercise program, start by exercising around 65 percent of your maximum heart rate. As you become more conditioned, increase your intensity gradually to 70 percent of your maximum heart rate. Then, after a few more weeks, increase to 75 percent, and so on. You may never be able to exercise at 85 percent of your maximum heart rate, especially if you are huffing and puffing. Remember: be sure that as you increase the intensity of your workouts, you remain able to converse with another person. That's the easiest way to ensure that you are working out at an intensity level that is healthy for you.

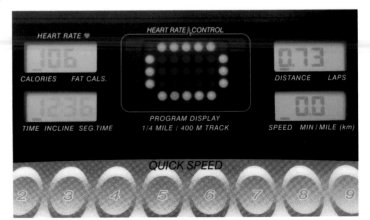

Calculating Your Target Heart Rate Zone

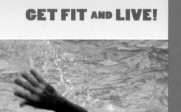

To calculate the low end of your target heart rate zone, start by subtracting your age from 220. This is your maximum heart rate. For example, if you are forty years old:

220 − 40 = 180 beats per minute

Now multiply this number by 65 percent to find the low end of your target heart rate zone.

180 x 0.65 = 117 beats per minute

To figure out the high end of your zone, multiply your maximum heart rate by 85 percent.

180 x 0.85 = 153 beats per minute

This means if you are forty, you should keep your heart rate between 117 and 153 beats per minute when exercising. Initially try and keep your heart rate around 117 to 125. Gradually increase your intensity, but make sure that you are able to converse while exercising and you are not huffing and puffing.

Exercise Within the Zone

Unless you have already been exercising consistently, I suggest that you initially set a goal of twenty minutes of exercise or activity a day, which may be split into ten minutes, twice a day. (You can do this by simply walking your dog!) Once you have adapted to that time, then you can gradually increase to thirty minutes and eventually forty minutes or longer. To minimize soreness, begin by doing exercises three days a week every other day to start with, and then work up to five or even six days a week . And remember, a brisk walk can accomplish almost the same thing as jogging, provided your maximum heart rate is maintained at 65 to 85 percent. The key is staying within your target heart rate zone and being able to carry on a conversation, which, again, usually ensures you are training at a healthy pace.

Dr. Colbert Approved

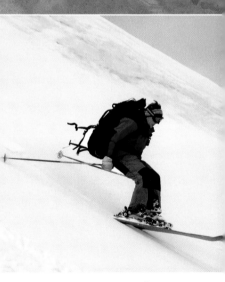

How Many Calories Are Burned During Activity?

Low Activity Level
Sleeping = 55 calories per hour
Eating = 85 calories per hour
Sewing = 85 calories per hour
Sitting = 85 calories per hour
Standing = 100 calories per hour
Driving = 110 calories per hour
Office work = 140 calories per hour

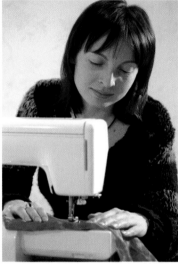

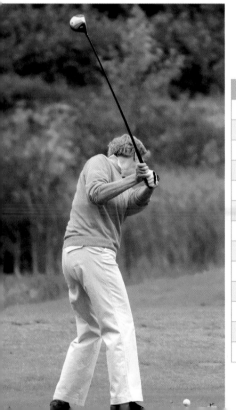

Moderate Activity Level
Housework, moderate = 160+ calories per hour
Golf, with golf cart = 180 calories per hour
Golf, with no golf cart = 240 calories per hour
Gardening, planting = 250 calories per hour
Dancing, ballroom = 260 calories per hour
Walking, 3 mph = 280 calories per hour
Ping-Pong = 290 calories per hour
Tennis = 350+ calories per hour
Water aerobics = 400 calories per hour
Skating/Rollerblading = 420+ calories per hour
Dancing, aerobic = 420+ calories per hour
Aerobics = 450+ calories per hour
Bicycling, moderate = 450+ calories per hour

High Activity Level
Jogging, 5 mph = 500 calories per hour
Gardening, digging = 500 calories per hour
Swimming, active = 500+ calories per hour
Hiking = 500+ calories per hour
Step aerobics = 550+ calories per hour
Rowing = 550+ calories per hour
Power walking = 600+ calories per hour
Cycling, studio = 650 calories per hour
Squash = 650+ calories per hour
Skipping rope = 700+ calories per hour
Running = 700+ calories per hour

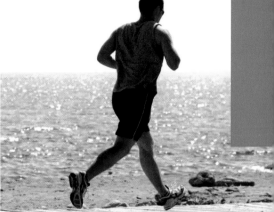

Fidgeting as Exercise?

According to researchers at Mayo Clinic in Rochester, Minnesota, some people burn hundreds of calories every day . . . by fidgeting. Fidgeting includes crossing or uncrossing your legs, bobbing up and down, stretching or standing up often, or being generally restless.

Researchers fed subjects one thousand extra calories per day for eight weeks. As a result, some subjects automatically began fidgeting to burn the extra calories. About 33 percent of the one thousand extra calories consumed were burned by fidgeting and restlessness. Of the remaining calories, approximately 39 percent were deposited as fat. The participants gained from two to sixteen pounds, but the most fidgety people gained the least amount of fat.[1]

Put another way, fidgeting or getting up from your seat frequently can cause you to burn an additional 330 calories a day— which amounts to 36 pounds lost in a year!

The "Real" Price Tag on That Cookie

If you're thinking about grabbing an unhealthy snack, think again. Here are the calorie contents of popular snack foods and the amount of time it would take you to burn those calories by brisk walking (which burns about 8 calories per minute).

- Chips Ahoy, 3 cookies (240 calories) = 30 minutes
- Oreos, 3 cookies (169 calories) = about 20 minutes
- Glazed doughnut, 4 oz. (400 calories) = 50 minutes
- Ritz crackers, original, 6 oz. serving (80 calories) = 10 minutes
- Burger King Whopper (670 calories) = 1 hour and 30 minutes
- Baked Doritos Nacho Cheesier, 10 chips (80 calories) = 10 minutes
- Lay's Classic potato chips, 10 chips (80 calories) = 10 minutes

5

WHAT KIND OF EXERCISE DO YOU NEED?

Key Components of a Good Workout

EVERY FITNESS PROGRAM NEEDS to include the following key components: (1) some form of aerobic activity, (2) some form of anaerobic activity (muscle building or toning), and (3) warming up and cooling down with proper stretching for proper posture and flexibility.

Aerobic means "in the presence of air." It's the kind of exercise that gets you breathing deeply and more rapidly than normal. Aerobic exercises generally work the large muscle groups of the body in repetitive motions for a sustained period of time. We'll discuss more about this later in the chapter.

Anaerobic means "without air" and refers to short, higher-intensity workouts. Working out with weights and performing calisthenics are the most effective ways to get fit through anaerobic activity. We'll give you more information on anaerobic exercise later in this chapter.

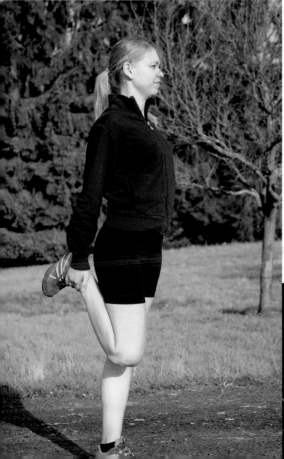

Last but certainly not least, flexibility and posture are extremely important components of a good workout, which is why we've devoted two chapters of this book to them. Stretches are the primary way you improve your posture and flexibility. See chapter 7 for more information on cooling down with the proper stretches.

For the remainder of this chapter, we'll focus on the two basic categories of exercise—aerobic and anaerobic—and the various activities you can choose for each category.

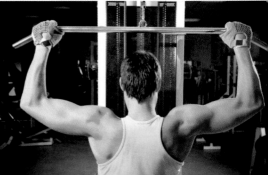

Step 1: Get a Checkup

We can't repeat it often enough—the first thing to do before you begin any fitness program is to have your physician give you a thorough exam. Nobody should start a fitness program until they know their body can handle it. It's also a good idea to have an EKG and a stress test to ensure you have a healthy heart. Your heart is a muscle, and it must be conditioned gradually and consistently—like all your muscles—to reach its optimum performance. Don't try to run a five-mile race or a marathon tomorrow if you have been a couch potato for the last five years. It will do more harm than good! The American College of Sports Medicine recommends a medical examination and exercise testing prior to participation in vigorous exercise for all male adults over forty-five and all females over fifty-five.

Step 2: Keep It Simple— and Smart!

Once you have been examined, it's time to get started. Keep it simple and fun—like walking—to get you started. But don't forget to keep it smart. Use your head when you work out. Never exercise without addressing your posture and flexibility by warming up with the proper stretches, and always practice mindful exercising.

Dr. Colbert Approved

Exercise Program

There are three components to a good fitness program:

- Aerobic exercise, such as brisk walking

- Anaerobic exercise (strengthening and toning exercises), such as weight lifting and calisthenics

- Flexibility and posture exercises, such as stretching

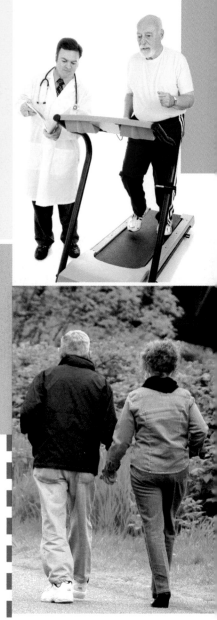

Types of Aerobic Exercise

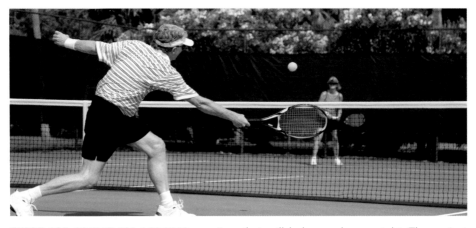

THERE ARE COUNTLESS AEROBIC exercises that will help you lose weight. The easiest activity, as I just mentioned, is taking a brisk walk. I am not referring to a leisurely stroll but rather a lively, relatively fast-paced walk. Other good aerobic activities include bike riding (either on a stationary bike or a real one), jogging slowly, aerobic dancing, hiking, cardio yoga, and using an elliptical machine or stair stepper. Sports such as basketball, volleyball, soccer, football, racquetball, tennis, and squash are all considered aerobic exercises. Pilates, ballroom dancing, washing the car by hand, working in your yard, and mowing the grass are other activities within this category. Swimming and water aerobics are also good aerobic exercises, but unless done as sport (rather than leisure) they often do not burn as much fat as other forms of exercise.

The key is finding something that you enjoy and that you will do on a regular basis four to six days a week. For some of you, that may be playing hoops with your children when you get home from work. For others, it may be as simple as walking your dog thirty minutes a day.

Remember, you do not have to exercise vigorously to burn fat. Too many of us think that we have to suffer and sweat to burn fat, but that is simply not the case. A simple rule of thumb is to walk slow enough so that you can talk but fast enough so that you cannot sing. If you are walking and singing, then speed it up; but if you are unable to carry on a conversation while walking, then slow it down. You may want to purchase a heart rate monitor so you can adjust your exercise intensity to enter and stay in the fat-burning range. These can be purchased at most sporting goods stores, while most cardio equipment at health clubs are already equipped with them.

Exercising with a buddy greatly improves compliance and usually adds enjoyment to the activity. We encourage people to get an activity buddy, such as a spouse, friend, neighbor, or child.

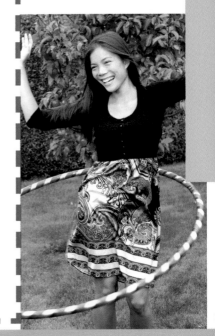

Dr. Colbert Approved

Aerobic Exercises

- Most adults: Engage in at least thirty minutes of moderate-intensity physical activity, above usual activity, at work or home on most days of the week.

- Children and adolescents: Engage in at least sixty minutes of physical activity on most, preferably all, days of the week.

- Pregnant women: In the absence of medical or obstetric complications, incorporate thirty minutes or more of moderate-intensity physical activity on most days of the week.

- Older adults: Participate in regular physical activity to reduce functional declines associated with aging.[1]

Climb Your Way to a Longer Life

One Harvard study revealed a 23 percent higher mortality risk and a 56 percent higher coronary heart disease risk in men who climbed fewer than twenty flights of stairs per week than those who climbed more. If you live in a two-story home, be sure to climb the stairs at least a few times per day in order to meet the minimum twenty flights per week you need to reap these benefits.[2]

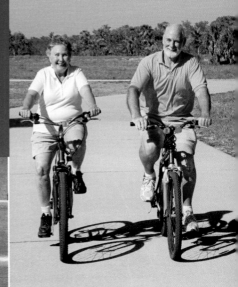

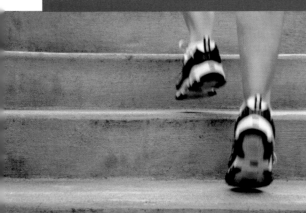

As Simple as a Brisk Walk

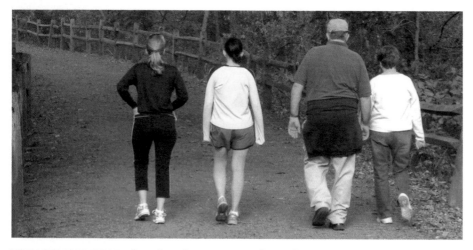

YOU MIGHT BE TIRED of reading this recommendation, but it is the truth! Brisk walking is one of the best aerobic exercises we can recommend, and it's virtually free. It can give you three times the normal amount of oxygen you would otherwise get. Buy a good pair of walking shoes so you don't injure your feet, and find a soft walking surface so you don't injure your joints. Walk slowly enough so that you can talk, but walk fast enough so that you can't sing. Window-shopping doesn't count. Keep a steady pace without stopping.

One woman we know started walking briskly four times a week for thirty minutes, and after one year she had lost eighty pounds. "What about your diet?" we asked her.

"I didn't change my eating habits at all," she said.

Not bad results for a regular walk around the block!

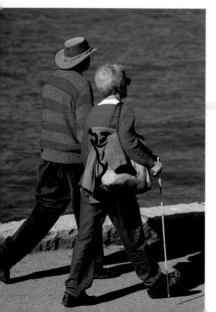

Make Sure the Air in Your Aerobic Workout Is *Fresh* Air!

Choose your location wisely. Walking or jogging by a busy highway is almost worse than sitting at home eating bonbons. We often see people jogging by the side of the road during high traffic, and not ten feet away buses and trucks go by pumping out big plumes of diesel exhaust. Those pollutants go into every cell in your body, and it's difficult to get rid of some of them.

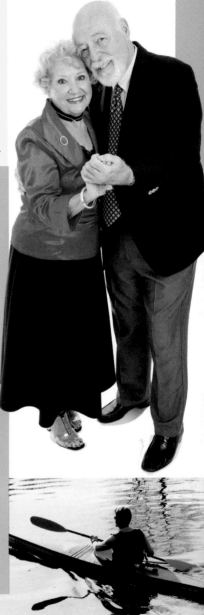

Quick Quiz

A 160-pound person burns this many calories per minute while walking briskly (5 mph):

(a) 8.7 calories per minute

(b) 15 calories per minute

(c) 2.1 calories per minute

Answer: a. 8.7 calories per minute. Slower walking (2 mph) burns only 3.4 calories per minute—less than half that of brisk walking.[3]

Aerobics at a Glance

Walking is a form of aerobic exercise. Other forms of aerobic exercises include:

- Jogging
- Cycling
- Rowing
- Elliptical machine or glider
- Aerobic dance routines
- Stair stepping
- Skating
- Cross-country skiing
- Singles tennis
- Racquetball
- Basketball
- Ballroom dancing or other forms of dance
- Swimming

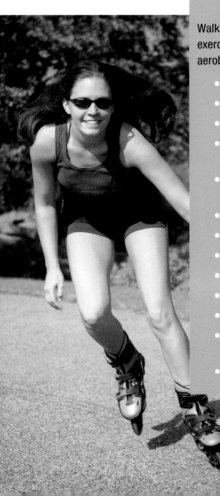

ANAEROBIC EXERCISE

AS WE'VE JUST EXPLAINED, aerobic exercise is great for the heart and lungs. However, it's also important to strengthen your bones and muscles through anaerobic exercise. Weight training and calisthenics are the two common ways to add anaerobic exercise to your fitness routine. Beginning at age thirty, everyone needs to exercise either with weights or calisthenics to keep their muscles and bones strong and avoid diseases associated with aging, such as osteoporosis.

On these two pages, we'll help you understand how to easily add a weight-lifting program to your fitness routine. On the next two pages, we'll address calisthenics.

Working With Weights

Here are ten tips we'd like to offer you for working with weights:

- Start each workout with stretching followed by an aerobic warm-up of five to ten minutes to get blood flowing to your muscles. This will decrease your chance of injury.

- Next, find a weight that you can lift for at least eight, but not more than twelve, repetitions. (Remember, low-intensity workouts reduce your risk of injury and muscle strain, so easy does it.)

- You should be training at about 60 percent of your maximum ability. Perform each repetition slowly, using good control. (We'll discuss more about this in chapter 7, when we explain the concept of mindful exercising.)

- You can perform more than one set of repetitions, but if you are just beginning a weight-lifting routine you should rest for at least a minute or two between working the same muscle group. In time, you will only need to rest thirty seconds to a minute between repetitions.

- The heavier the weight you are lifting, the fewer repetitions you should attempt. Heavier weights with low repetitions improve muscular strength.

- Lighter weights with high repetitions (more than twelve repetitions) build muscular endurance and tone the muscles. Moderate weights with moderate repetitions do both.

- As your strength increases over the weeks, you may increase the amount of weight you lift by no more than 5 percent each workout. We recommend training using moderate weights and moderate repetitions (eight to twelve repetitions) to avoid injury.

- Ideally you should work out with weights three days per week with a day between workouts.

- We find that it's helpful—and safer—to lift weights with a friend once you get going. It also keeps you accountable to someone so you are less likely to miss a workout.

- Initially, working on a weight machine is safer than working with free weights because you are less likely to injure yourself.

Benefits of Weight Lifting[4]

Here are some of the benefits of weight lifting:

- Increases muscle mass
- Elevates your metabolism, which helps burn fat
- Improves posture
- Provides better support for joints
- Reduces the risk of injury from everyday activities
- Reverses the loss of muscle tissue that normally accompanies aging
- Helps to prevent osteoporosis
- Increases levels of dopamine, serotonin, and norepinephrine, which can help to improve mood and counter feelings of depression

Quick Quiz

True or false: If you don't feel pain, you're not lifting enough weight.

Answer: False. If you feel pain, you are generally lifting too much weight and/or doing too many repetitions. You should feel resistance and should strain a bit, but pain itself is a sign you are going beyond your abilities and may injure yourself.

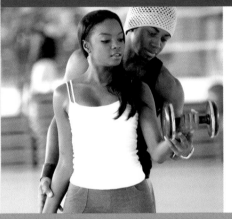

Benefits of a Certified Personal Trainer

If you can afford it, we highly recommend that you find a certified personal trainer to train you in the correct form and technique. He or she can get you started on the right program, help you avoid injury, and teach you flexibility and stretching exercises too.

Additionally, a certified trainer will help you exercise your eight to ten different muscle groups, including the chest, back, shoulders, arms, abdomen, upper and lower back, and legs and calves. He or she will help you to maintain proper form, work your full range of motion, provide movtivation and accountability, and teach you proper breathing during exercises.

Practicing Mindfulness During Weight Lifting

PRACTICING MINDFULNESS IS EXTREMELY important while exercising, especially with lifting weights or performing calisthenic or resistance band exercises. It's not as important to practice mindfulness with aerobic exercises such as walking, jogging, cycling, and swimming because you can let your mind wander or watch TV while on the treadmill and still get the benefits of aerobic exercise. But when it comes to weight lifting, calisthenics, or resistance band exercises, we have found that it is critically important to practice mindfulness or you will simply not reap the full benefit of these exercises.

Mindful exercise—or more specifically, mindful lifting—is similar to the concept of mindful eating, which is discussed in more detail in *Eat This and Live!* and *Dr. Colbert's "I Can Do This" Diet*. When you practice mindful eating, you savor the taste of food and are aware of how much you are eating.

Conversely, mind*less* eating is when you stop paying attention to the taste or amount of food you are eating and eat on autopilot while watching TV, talking on the phone, or working on the computer. Mindless lifting is when people are exercising on autopilot and not focused on their posture, on using correct form and lifting techniques, on performing the movement slowing while engaging the muscles, or on proper breathing.

Both of us work out at a gym on a regular basis, and it amazes us to look around and see that more than 95 percent of the people working out—even those working with personal trainers—are not practicing mindful lifting. They are putting hours in the gym each week, probably paying big bucks, but ending up with little to show for it because of the mindlessness of their workouts. If you've never been to a gym, the sidebar on mindless lifting on the next page will explain what we often see.

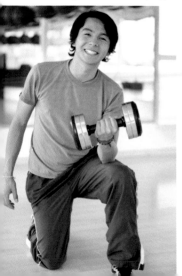

Definition, Please...

Renowned cardiologist Herbert Benson defined *mindfulness* as "the practice of learning to pay attention to what is happening to you from moment to moment. To be mindful, you must slow down, do one activity at a time, and bring your full awareness to both the activity at hand and to your inner experience of it." Mindfulness means simply to let go of any thought that is unrelated to the present moment and to find something to enjoy in the present.

Mindless Lifting

These are the things we see in the gym every day
that reveal mindlessness when it comes to weight training:

- People on the bench press lifting the weight rapidly and bouncing the bar off their chest; they usually perform semi reps and never fully engage their muscles.

- People performing barbell curls on autopilot; they almost always display poor posture with their shoulders rounded as they begin to curl the weight.

- People bringing their elbows up as they do barbell curls; this prevents them from working the entire biceps.

- People using their lower back to help to swing the weight up; after they have curled the barbell up, they let it drop and repeat this very poor lifting technique.

This mindless lifting is not engaging the muscles properly; it is stressing muscles and tendons since the posture is compromised, and it is setting them up for eventual injury.

Mindful Lifting

Dr. Colbert Approved

Now let's see how to practice mindful lifting.

- First make sure your posture is correct with your shoulders back, chest out, waist in, and your head over your shoulders.

- Keep your core (abs) tight while performing all exercises.

- When doing curls, keep the tension on the biceps while curling throughout the entire movement as you perform the movement slowly, keeping the bicep muscles engaged.

- Continue to flex the biceps as you lower the barbell slowly, keeping the biceps again fully engaged.

- Perform eight to twelve repetitions, and do about three sets.

- Concentrate on breathing and flexing the biceps while performing the exercise, and do not let your mind wander.

- My exercise program is usually very quick, and I finish my weight training in about twenty or thirty minutes and then go on to cardio.

- I have also learned that if I close my eyes during my exercises, I have even less distractions and am able to focus better.

By combining mindful lifting with muscle engagement, I have seen tremendous gains in my strength and muscle definition.

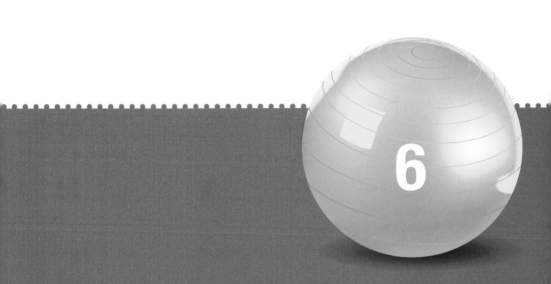

6

FUN, ALTERNATIVE FITNESS

YOGA

MANY PEOPLE DON'T ENJOY traditional exercises like the ones we've been talking about, but they do enjoy alternative exercises that help stir the waters of their body with motion. In this chapter we'll cover some of the most helpful—and fun—alternative exercises. On this page, we'll discuss yoga, followed by tai chi, Pilates, and other fun fitness alternatives on the remaining pages of the chapter.

Yoga has been shown to decrease tension, stress, anxiety, depression, and hypertension. People who do a form of yoga called Sahaja show improvement in blood pressure, heart rate, levels of blood lactate, levels of the stress hormone epinephrine in the urine, and the galvanic skin resistance test, which indicates whether the patient is tense or relaxed.[1]

Yoga is different from most other forms of exercise in that it is not concerned with how many repetitions are performed or how well a person performs a particular exercise. Instead, yoga focuses your attention on how your body is structured and how to move without aggravating an injury or causing pain. It teaches you to breathe properly and to integrate breathing with positions of the body. You don't strain or force your body when doing yoga, but rather gently stretch various muscles. It feels terrific! It improves your strength, flexibility, and endurance. In fact, one study in the *Journal of the American Medical Association* reported that daily yoga practice could reduce the pain associated with carpal tunnel syndrome.[2]

If you are concerned with flexibility and learning to understand your various muscle groups through low-impact exercise, yoga is probably your best option.

Types of Yoga

There are several types of yoga. Hatha yoga is the most popular type practiced in the United States. It concentrates on controlled breathing and posture. The slow breathing promotes relaxation, and the various postures of hatha yoga promote flexibility by gently stretching the body into different positions.

Other forms of yoga include ashtanga, or power yoga, generally preferred by athletes to develop strength and stamina. Bikram yoga is done in a hot room that is 100 degrees Fahrenheit or higher, and it is recommended only for extremely fit individuals. There are several other forms of yoga beyond these.

Is Yoga OK for Christians?

We are sometimes asked if we feel it is acceptable for Christians to promote the practice of yoga. The answer is, we only promote the physical exercises of yoga, never its spiritual or Eastern meditative aspects. We feel that it is possible to ignore the spiritual baggage and religious associations that are often associated with yoga and still enjoy terrific, low-impact exercise that combines stretching and breathing to relax the body.

Because we're Christians, when we do yoga, we meditate on Christ. We never encourage people to meditate on a mantra, but to meditate on the Scriptures or on the name of Jesus and His various attributes and titles in the Bible instead. I recommend finding a Christian yoga class, and I caution you to watch for Sanskrit language that pays tribute to Hindu deities, metaphysical/New Age jargon ("negative and positive energy," "divinity within you," "focus on the third eye," etc.), and projection (emptying your mind or stepping outside your body). If you feel uncomfortable in any way, it might be God's way of telling you that a yoga class is not right for you. If that is the case, consider the other alternatives for exercise that we explain throughout this chapter.

TAI CHI

TAI CHI IS AN ancient Chinese martial art that involves slow, smooth, fluid movements. It emphasizes diaphragmatic or abdominal breathing. Its movements are smooth, graceful, low intensity, and accompanied by rhythmic abdominal breathing. A typical exercise session is a series of gentle, deliberate movements or postures combined into a sequential "choreography." These series of movements are called forms, and each form is comprised of a series of twenty to one hundred tai chi movements. Each form can take up to twenty minutes to complete. Tai chi relies totally on technique rather than power or strength.

Various Health Benefits of Tai Chi [3]

Research has shown that tai chi may improve muscle mass, tone, flexibility, strength, stamina, balance, coordination, posture, and well-being. It can also give similar cardiovascular benefits to modern aerobic exercise. People who practice tai chi report less tension, depression, anger, fatigue, confusion, and anxiety, and feel more vigorous.

Meditate on God's Word

Tai chi lowers stress hormones, increases energy, and helps clear the mind. You can do it at any age, even if you have a chronic disease or health problem. Tai chi calms the mind, promotes flexibility, and exercises and tones the body, including the cardiovascular system. Like yoga, it includes meditation. I believe this is a great opportunity to meditate on God's Word!

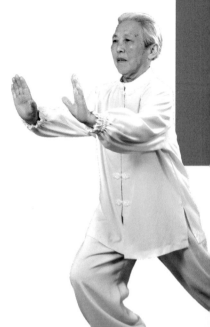

GET FIT AND LIVE!

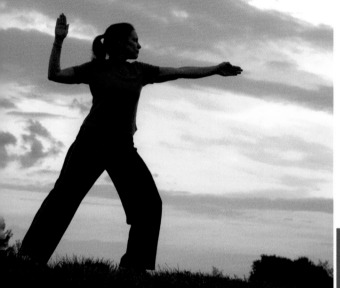

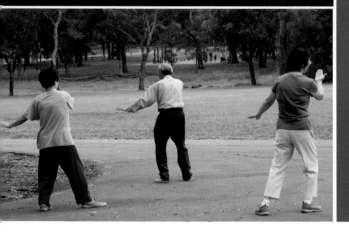

Tai Chi for Arthritis[4]

Tai chi is an exceptionally good exercise for older people who have arthritis, peripheral vascular disease, chronic obstructive pulmonary disease, osteoporosis, or other physical problems. The Arthritis Foundation recommends tai chi for individuals with arthritis.

PILATES

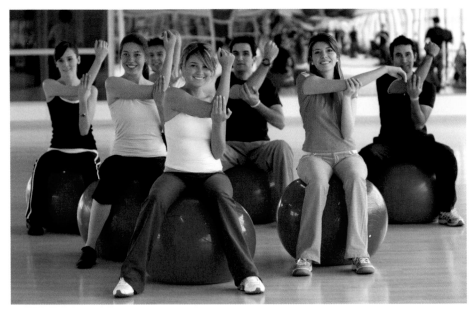

PILATES EXERCISES WERE DEVELOPED by Joseph Pilates in the early twentieth century. As a child, Joseph suffered from rheumatic fever, rickets, and asthma. He was determined to overcome his ailments, and he began studying anatomy at a young age. During World War II, he worked as a nurse and developed equipment to help rehabilitate the war injured. He would take bedsprings and attach them to the ceiling so that bedridden patients might exercise and gain strength. Eventually he opened an exercise studio in New York City, where he trained many great dancers.[5]

Instead of performing many repetitions of each exercise, Pilates preferred fewer, more precise movements, requiring control and form. He designed more than five hundred specific exercises. The most frequent form, called "mat work," involves a series of calisthenic motions performed without weights or apparatus on a padded mat. Pilates believed that mental health and physical health were essential to one another. He created what is claimed to be a method of total body conditioning that emphasizes proper alignment, centering, concentration, control, precision, breathing, and flowing movement (the Pilates principles) that result in increased flexibility, strength, muscle tone, body awareness, energy, and improved mental concentration.[6] Pilates also helps to reduce tension and stress. Many health clubs now offer Pilates exercise classes.

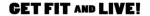

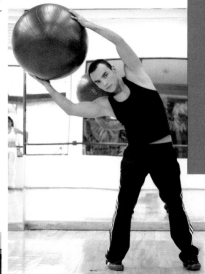

The Six Principles of Pilates

1. Centering: this principle involves focusing on the center of the body, the abdomen.

2. Concentration: this principle involves concentrating on each exercise for maximum value to be obtained from each movement.

3. Control: this principle teaches you to conduct each movement with complete muscular control.

4. Precision: this principle emphasizes awareness of the appropriate placement, alignment, and trajectory of each part of the body during movement.

5. Breath: Pilates exercises coordinate movement with proper breathing.

6. Flow: this principle emphasizes fluidity, grace, and ease as goals of exercise.

MORE FUN, ALTERNATIVE FITNESS IDEAS

Ballroom Dancing

BALLROOM DANCING IS AN excellent alternative for anyone who does not enjoy exercising but does enjoy dancing! It provides most benefits of aerobic exercise without the feeling that you are exercising. It is low-impact aerobic exercise that uses the large muscle groups of the body. It can be done for thirty minutes or for an entire evening.

Ballroom dancing can help you develop coordination, balance, and rhythm. It is usually associated with a very pleasant environment, with soothing music, and with an opportunity for creative expression and social interaction. Among the more common dances are the fox-trot, swing, cha-cha, tango, waltz, rumba, mambo, samba, and merengue.

People who become bored with treadmills or exercise bikes usually find ballroom dancing a fun alternative. Classes are often offered at a college, university, or private studio. The basic steps for most dances can be learned from videos, DVDs, or books. An inexpensive way to explore the possibility of doing ballroom dancing is to rent or buy a basic dance video.

Ballroom dancing is also a great way for married couples to reconnect. It's a great way to spend time together and exercise at the same time!

Passive Exercise

In addition to a fitness program that includes all of the key ingredients we discussed in the last chapter, we believe in something we call "passive exercise." Intentionally forgoing the following modern conveniences allows you to capitalize on common exercise opportunities many people miss:

- Park in the farthest parking space from your destination and walk the extra distance.

- If your destination is less than a mile from your home, consider walking or riding a bike instead of driving.

- Take the stairs instead of the elevator or escalator.

- Rake the leaves or shovel snow instead of using a leaf or snow blower.

- Walk to a co-worker's office or cubicle when communication is necessary instead of calling or e-mailing.

Some Sports Video Games and Fitness Packages Burn as Many Calories as the Real Thing[7]

WebMD.com recently reported that some Wii sports video games burn as many calories as moderate-intensity exercises like brisk walking. A study funded by Nintendo found that about a third of the games in Wii sports video and fitness packages require the same energy expenditure as moderate-intensity exercise.

Twelve men and women, ages twenty-five to forty-four, were measured while performing the basic moves of Wii sports games and fitness programs. You might be surprised by the results: twenty-three of the games required an energy expenditure of 2 to 3 METs, which borders on the American Heart Association's definition of moderate-intensity exercise. (See the "What's an MET?" sidebar on this page for more information.)

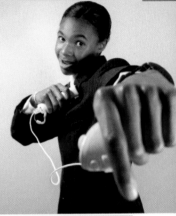

The highest intensity "virtual" exercise was the single-arm stand in the Wii Fit, which came in at almost 6 METs. Second place went to the Wii sports boxing game at 4.5 METs, while both the Wii tennis and baseball games produced moderate-intensity expenditures of about 3 METs (the equivalent of brisk walking in the "real world").

While we believe that getting out and involving yourself in real physical activity is still the best way to get fit, this research shows that any form of physical activity, even the video variety, is better than none. Since this chapter is dedicated to fun alternative forms of fitness, we felt it was worth mentioning this entertaining new way to increase your activity level.

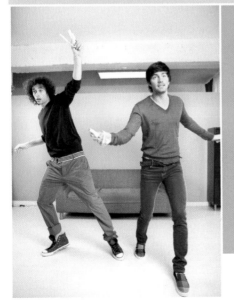

What's an MET?

The researchers who conducted the Wii sports video games study used a standard method of measuring energy expenditure called METs, or metabolic equivalent values. According to exercise guidelines from the American Heart Association (AHA), activity that expends fewer than 3 METs is considered light-intensity, activity using 3 to 6 METs is considered moderate intensity, and vigorous activity is measured at more than 6 METs. For example, according to the AHA, an adult who walks briskly (at a pace of 3 miles an hour) on a flat surface expends a little more than 3 METs.

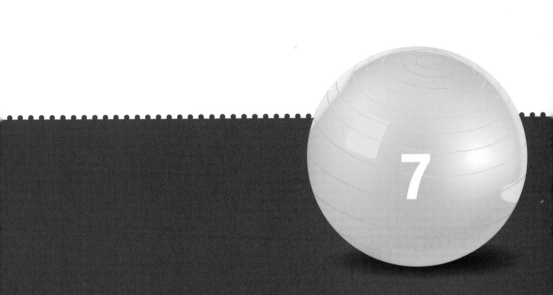

THE IMPORTANCE OF CORRECT POSTURE

IS YOUR POOR POSTURE SHOWING?

OVER THE YEARS, I have discovered that my healthiest patients were usually those who maintained good posture. Good posture is also critically important to maintain while exercising. However, most individuals have poor posture and continue to exercise with poor posture, which in turn may actually worsen their posture. They also do not get the most important benefits of their exercise regimen due to poor posture. Incorporating the postural exercises to your workout program actually retrains your postural muscles and improves your exercise form, and in turn, you reap greater benefits while following your exercise program.

Posture also tells quite a lot of information about a person. For example, an exhausted person will usually slouch forward with rounded shoulders, and their head is forward and down. I can typically spot a depressed person from over 100 yards away because they have unique posture. The depressed person also has slouch-rounded shoulders. Their shoulders are drawn down and forward typically. The head is low and usually hanging down. They move slowly and sort of drag along. Depression is literally written all over their body. Unfortunately, I now see the tired and exhausted posture as well as depression posture commonly in teens as well as adults. They actually look like they have been beaten down and carry the burden of the world on their shoulders.

However, someone who is joyful, energetic, and confident usually holds their head high and centered over their shoulders; they also hold their spine erect with their shoulders back. They typically move with energy and vitality and usually have passion for life. Their posture literally exudes confidence, energy, vitality, and joy.

I have found that I can teach my patients how to develop good posture, and with practice, good posture can eventually become a habit in their lives. What is encouraging is that as my tired and depressed patients continue to practice proper posture, many are able to experience energy, vitality, and confidence once more. I will never forget the patient of mine who was seventy-five years old and suffered from many diseases and was taking many different medications. Her diseases included fibromyalgia, chronic fatigue, arthritis, hypertension, high cholesterol, and type 2 diabetes. Her husband, who was eighty years old, would bring her to the office, and what was so odd was that he had no pain, no chronic diseases, and he took no medication. I also noticed that his posture commanded respect. He was eighty years old with perfect posture like a marine at attention. He maintained that posture as he sat, stood, and walked. His shoulders were broad, his spine was erect, his head was held high and centered over his shoulders, his chest was out, and his abdomen was in. Most elderly men that I see have rounded shoulders, their head is forward like a turtle's head, their chest is sunken in, their belly protruded out, and their bottom is tucked in. Unfortunately, this man's wife was suffering from many diseases, but she also had very poor posture. I asked him how he was able to maintain such excellent posture at his age, and he simply smiled and said that since he was a boy, his mom and dad had hounded him on his posture. You see, he also used to slouch, but with practicing good posture, it had eventually become a habit. Now he does not even have to think about it. On the other hand, his wife developed a habit of poor posture. Unfortunately, her parents did not hound her about her poor posture and let her do as she pleased. As a result, she did what was comfortable and eventually developed many diseases, some of which may be related to her poor posture.

Sleeping Instructions

I recommend my patients sleep on their sides or their back, rather than sleeping on their stomach. Make sure you have a comfortable mattress. However, I have found that a three-inch Tempur-Pedic pad on top of a mattress is great for back support. Make sure you have a comfortable and not overstuffed pillow to provide support for the head and neck.

The Effect of Gravity on Posture

As we get older, our bodies naturally begin to sag, and our posture gradually erodes as aging and gravity literally pull us forward and down. The head goes forward instead of being centered over the shoulders where it belongs. As a result, many older individuals look like they have a turtle head with the head jutting outward instead of centered over the shoulders. In many third world countries, small women have been able to carry loads of thirty pounds or more by simply maintaining good posture and keeping their head positioned over their shoulders. According to Psalm 139:14, we are fearfully and wonderfully made. God has created the human neck and spine similar to a scaffolding system with three unique curves. This unique scaffold enables us to stand erect because the spine is shaped similarly to an elongated S with three unique curves—the cervical, thoracic, and lumbar curves. The spine S curve is the centerpiece of the scaffold; however, there are also four key load-bearing joints on each side of the body, including the shoulders, hips, knees, and ankles, which need to be aligned and balanced. Muscles then move the bones by contracting and relaxing. Our bodies were meant for motion. However, unfortunately many people's scaffolding is sagging so that movement may not be comfortable or is in fact painful for them. Their shoulders are usually rounded, head protruding forward, their pelvis is usually forward, and the S curve of the spine has been in flexion for so long that it starts to look more like a C or an inverted J curve. Our muscles and bones are fighting gravity, and gravity is winning. However, by practicing unique postural exercises, stretching and stretching exercises, we restore posture and build strong, flexible muscles.

Tires

Poor posture is very similar to driving your car with your tires out of alignment. Over time you eventually wear down your tires unevenly, and eventually the car will ride rough or steer poorly. Over time you may get a knot on the tire (similar to a bulging disk), or tire blowout (similar to a herniated disk), or worn out tires (similar to a degenerative disk). Are you beginning to get the picture?

FINDING YOUR CORRECT POSTURE

NOW THAT YOU HAVE heard all of the hazards of poor posture, let me show you how to find the correct posture for your body. Ask a friend to take a photo of you from the side. Men should remove their shirts, and women should wear a bra or swim suit. Stand up as you normally would; relax as though you are not thinking about your posture. Now look at your photograph. The middle of your ear should be aligned with the middle of your shoulder, the middle of your hip, the middle of your knee, and the middle of your ankle. Remember the four load-bearing joints that make up the unique scaffold of your body. It is important that this be aligned in order for you to maintain correct posture. This is especially important when you exercise. If you are unable to draw a straight line through these areas of your body, then you need to perform postural exercises on a daily basis. Realize that over time, poor posture takes a major toll on the joints of the neck, spine, shoulders, hips, knees, and ankles. This may eventually lead to joint pain, arthritis, degeneration, muscle strains and sprains, muscle imbalance, decreased flexibility, decreased strength, weight gain, and other diseases.

Learning, practicing, and maintaining good posture is absolutely vital for the success of your exercise program. Unfortunately, I have not heard of any doctors or personal trainers who emphasize this. For the vast majority of Americans, poor posture is weakening their postural muscles to the extent that it is quite difficult for many to try to maintain good posture even for a minute. For some elderly people, they have been in a stooped position for so long that they are literally unable to stand up straight. I have seen many people that literally have to lie down in order to look up because they cannot extend their neck. The good thing is that practicing some key exercises can correct your posture. You will need to practice maintaining good posture while exercising, standing, sitting, and walking.

Incorrect   **Correct**

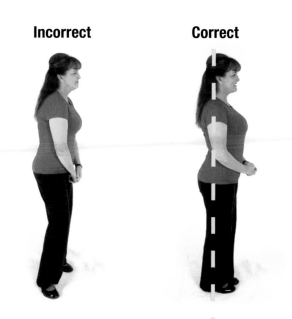

Do You Have a Turtlehead?

The average human head weighs approximately eight pounds. For every inch that the head moves forward and is not centered over the shoulders, it increases the weight of the head on the neck by approximately ten pounds. Therefore, the forward head posture of three inches increases the weight of the head on the neck by approximately thirty pounds, and it also increases the pressure on the muscle of the neck by about six times. The turtle head posture increases the weight of the head even more. Chronic forward head posture may eventually lead to long-term muscle strain on the neck, degenerative disk disease, arthritis, disk herniation, and pinched nerves.

Also, the shoulders slouch and drop as gravity and poor posture begin to pull them forward toward the ground. This stooped-over posture used to be seen mainly in the elderly, but now it is very common in teens and even children. Stooped posture even restricts our ability to take a deep breath, and as a result, one's energy level usually drops. Our bodies require adequate oxygen to function optimally, and slouched posture may be preventing you from obtaining adequate oxygen to feel energetic, refreshed, and revitalized.

Dr. Colbert Approved

The Correct Way to Lift Objects

Make it a habit to bend at the knees and not at the waist. Do not use your lower back for lifting, but instead use the leg muscles and stomach muscles. Always lift objects correctly by remembering the following rules:

1. While lifting, stand close to the object.

2. Never bend at the waist. Instead, bend your knees, keeping your back as straight as possible while maintaining the curvature (or lordosis) of your lower back.

3. Hold the object as close to your body as possible, and lift the object by straightening your knees. Maintain a steady motion; don't jerk the object.

4. Once you have assumed an upright position, do not twist the lower back. Turn by moving your feet.

The doctor of the future will give no medicine but will interest her or his patients in the care of the human frame, in a proper diet, and in the cause and prevention of disease.[1]

—Thomas A. Edison
U.S. Inventor (1847–1931)

POSTURE CORRECTION EXERCISES

Neck exercises for forward head posture

Stand with your back against the wall, heels six inches from the wall, buttocks touching the wall, and shoulders touching the wall. Now, gently pull your head back until it touches the wall while looking straight ahead. Pull your head back in this position for approximately five seconds. Perform four to five times. You should look similar to a turtle trying to pull its head back into the shell. You should not have any pain while performing this exercise, but if you do, consult your physician.

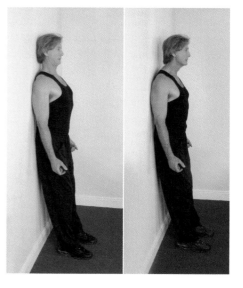

Postural correction of rounded shoulders

The shoulder blade squeeze: Stand with your elbows at your sides and your thumbs out like you are hitchhiking. Twist your forearms outward, and squeeze your shoulder blades together. Hold for five seconds, and perform four to five times during the day.

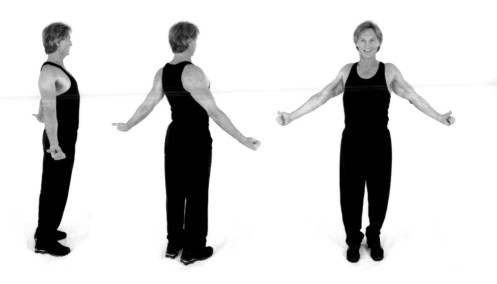

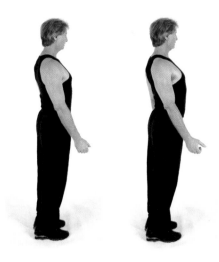

The breastbone lift: Stand and lift your breastbone a few inches higher, then pull your shoulder blades down and squeeze them together. Hold this position for five seconds, and perform four to five times during the day.

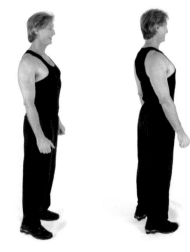

Postural exercises for the lower back

The lower back arch: Exaggerate the curve in the lower back. Hold for five seconds, and perform four to five times during the day.

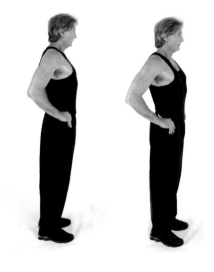

Tummy pull in: While inhaling, pull your tummy in and hold it tight, then exhale and keep your tummy tight. Hold for five seconds, and perform four to five times during the day.

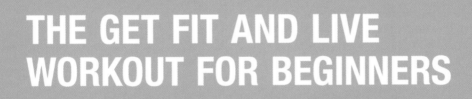

8

THE GET FIT AND LIVE WORKOUT FOR BEGINNERS

Important!

Before undergoing any activity or fitness program, please check with your doctor to make sure that you are healthy enough to participate.

IN THIS CHAPTER, WE'VE created three workouts for beginners. The plan is to give you a workout consisting of seven exercises that you can complete in seven minutes every Monday, Wednesday, and Friday. So when you turn the page, you'll see instructions and photos for the first exercise for Monday's workout. As the chapter progresses you'll learn how to do all seven exercises for Monday, Wednesday, and Friday.

Here are a few tips to help you make the most of your workout:

- **Timing:** To complete these workouts in seven minutes, your goal should be to perform each exercise for thirty seconds, and then either rest or rebound (jump on a minitrampoline) for thirty seconds before moving on to the next exercise. (For instructions on rebounding, see page 164–165.)

- **Before and after:** We recommend that you warm up with the seven-minute rebounding routine in chapter 16 before your workout, and that you cool down with stretches we've provided for you in chapter 10.

- **Equipment:** For the beginner workouts you'll need some light dumbbells, a resistance band, and a stabilizer ball. You'll also need a rebounder for the warm-up and thirty-second intervals between exercises.

- **Household items:** You'll need a sturdy chair, a phone book (optional), an ottoman or bench, and a door.

As a bonus for purchasing this book, we've made the videotaped demonstrations of several stretches and exercises we produced for *The Seven Pillars of Health* available to you. If you'd like to download this FREE twenty-minute video, visit www.sevenpillarsofhealth .com. NOTE: The video is not required for the workouts we're about to explain. It's additional coaching and instruction above and beyond what we've provided in this book. Some of the exercises and stretches in the video are the same as what you'll find on these pages, and some are different.

If you have special health conditions, before beginning your workout you should check with a doctor and read the remaining chapters of this book where we provide instruction for adapting these workouts to meet the special needs of those with diabetes, osteoporosis, arthritis, chronic fatigue, fibromyalgia, and more.

As you regularly perform these beginner workouts, your fitness will increase. After a few months you may be ready to move on to the intermediate and advanced workouts in chapter 9. Or you can simply increase the wieghts used on the beginner exercises. Some may even decide to contine the beginner exercises indefinitely because they do tone and strengthen muscles.

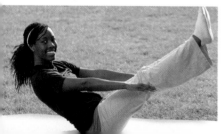

It's time to get fit and live! Are you ready? Turn the page, and let's get started!

Proper Breathing When Exercising

The most efficient oxygen exchange happens in your lower lungs, which is why deep breathing is so important. However, too many people practice shallow breathing. When you're exercising, it is especially important to avoid rapid, shallow breathing because this can cause dizziness and cramping. Improper breathing and especially holding your breath while lifting weights can also cause high blood pressure, fatigue, and overexertion.

To breathe properly, inhale slowly all the way down to your diaphragm (your belly should expand, not your chest), and then slowly exhale. If you are doing calisthenics or weight lifting with performed motions, exhaling on the exertion part of the exercise is considered the most beneficial way to breathe. For instance, when you do a sit-up, breathe out as you rise to a sitting position and inhale as you lie back down. But in general, if you focus on taking deep breaths without holding your breath, you'll avoid shallow breathing and fall into a comfortable pattern of breathing during exercise.

Dr. Colbert Approved

Definition, Please...

Repetitions, or *reps*, are simply how many times you perform a specific exercise. For example, "curls, eight repetitions" is simply the number of curls you perform, which is eight.

Set—a set is performed when a specified number of repetitions is performed for one particular exercise. The eight repetitions (or reps) of curls comprise one set. For beginners, I typically recommend starting off with one set of exercises for eight to twelve reps. As they become more conditioned, they can increase the number of sets to two or three sets per exercise. Beginners should still keep the reps consistent at eight to twelve, but as they become better conditioned, they can increase the amount of weight used. Remember, start low and go slow.

A good time to join a gym like Lifestyle Family Fitness is when you feel you are ready to advance to the intermediate workout.

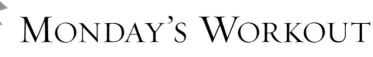

MONDAY'S WORKOUT

Target: Abdominals

Elbows to Knees

- Lie flat on the floor, keeping your lower back and head in contact with the floor, placing your hands on the side of your head. Lift both feet off the floor, keeping your ankles and knees together throughout the movement, while keeping your lower back pulled in to the floor.

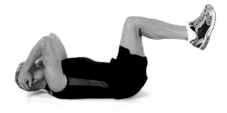

- Inhale and smoothly pull your knees toward your elbows. Avoid letting the legs come up or go out too far, as this can cause injury to the lower back.

- Squeezing a soft ball between your knees during the movement can make the exercise harder. Focus on keeping your abs contracted throughout, especially on the outward phase, where your feet should not touch the floor.

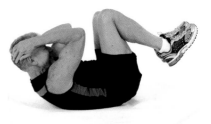

- Beginners aim for eight to twelve reps, not at full extension outward with the floor. Rest for twenty to thirty seconds. Initially do one set of eight to twelve reps but over time you may work up to two or three sets.

- When properly conditioned, instead of resting between sets, rebound for thirty seconds.

Caution!

Avoid the elbows-to-knees abdominal exercise if you suffer with lower-back problems.

MONDAY'S WORKOUT

Target: Core (Abdominals, Hips, and Back)

Plank

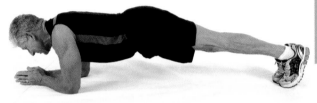

- Start by lying facedown on the ground, or use an exercise mat. Place your elbows and forearms underneath your chest. Prop yourself up to form a bridge using your toes and forearms. Maintain a flat back, and do not allow your hips to sag toward the ground.

- Hold this position and focus on tightening your abs until you can no longer maintain a flat bridge.

- Beginners should start with ten seconds, but over time eventually work up to thirty to sixty seconds.

Exactly What Is Your "Core"?

Your core is made up of about thirty muscles that wrap around your midsection (between your hips and ribs). These back muscles and deep abdominal muscles are key in supporting your spine and pelvis. Here are some things to remember about your core:

- Without awareness of your core as you exercise, you are more likely to experience back pain, injury, and posture problems.

- Contracting your core muscles (by simply drawing your belly button inward and holding for a few seconds) several times a day can do more to strengthen your core muscles than doing one hundred sit-ups!

- Remember to engage your core when you're exercising, playing sports, walking, or even sitting down, and you'll keep these muscles strong.

2

MONDAY'S WORKOUT

Target: Legs

Chair Squat

- Start off by standing two to four inches away from a chair with your back facing the chair. Stand with your feet shoulder width apart while crossing your arms in front of you.

- Bend your knees while keeping your shoulders and neck straight. Hover yourself one to two inches above the chair for two seconds, and stand up straight while keeping your knees slightly bent at standing position.

- Perform chair squats for eight to twelve reps.

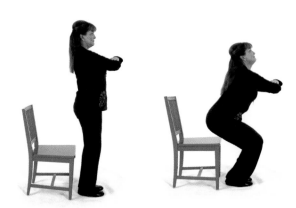

TIP: If you find this exercise too difficult at first, try placing a phone book on the chair (see photos).

- As this becomes easier, you can hold light dumbbells at shoulder level.

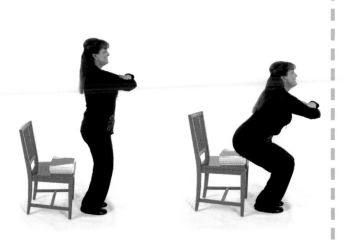

MONDAY'S WORKOUT

Target: Chest and Triceps

Ground Chest Press to Tricep Extension

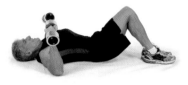

- Start out by lying on your back with your knees bent and feet flat on the floor. Keep your elbows away from your body while keeping elbows bent in a ninety-degree angle.

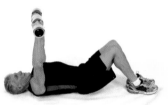

- Exhale through your mouth as you press the weights upward away from the body and bring the weights together.

- Rotate your hands inward, and keep your elbows tight (about ten inches away from each other), bending your elbows so that the weight will slowly move past your ears.

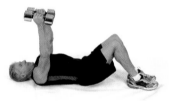

- Make a ninety-degree angle with your arms and hold for two seconds. Exhale and straighten your elbows until fully extended.

- Inhale through your nose as you release the weight back to the starting position with elbows on the ground.

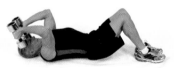

- Perform this exercise for eight to twelve repetitions.

If You Don't Have Dumbbells...

If you can't afford to purchase dumbbells, try using two full water bottles (20 oz. or larger) or two sacks of sugar. If the sugar is hard to hold on to, you can place each sack inside a plastic shopping bag and lift using the bag handles.

Monday's Workout

Target: Back

Arm Haulers

- Begin by laying flat on your stomach. Keep your arms extended above your head with your hands touching. Position your head facing down toward the ground to maintain good alignment of your neck and spine.

- The photo shows feet raised off the floor, but it is fine to let your feet touch the floor as you begin this exercise. You can lift your feet as your fitness increases.

- Slowly bring your arms around to your side while keeping your arms fully extended. (Think of doing a snow angel without moving your feet.) Remember not to hold your breath, but instead slowly feather your breathing as you bring your arms together over your head and back down to your sides.

- Perform this exercise for twenty seconds or eight to twelve repetitions (one repetition equals bringing your hands down to your sides and back together over your head).

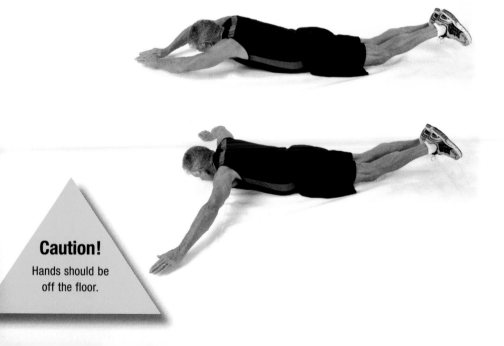

Caution!
Hands should be
off the floor.

Monday's Workout

Target: Arms and Biceps

Curls With Dumbbells or Resistance Bands

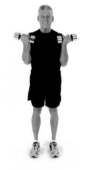

A. Dumbbells

- Position two dumbbells to sides, palms facing out, arms straight.

- With elbows to sides, raise one dumbbell and rotate forearm until forearm is vertical and palm faces shoulder.

- Lower to original position and perform with opposite arm. Continue to alternate between sides. Perform eight to twelve reps.

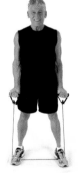 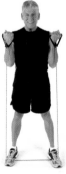

B. Resistance Bands

- Stand on the band and hold handles with palms facing out.

- Keeping abs in and knees slightly bent, bend arms and bring palms toward shoulders in a bicep curl.

- Position feet wider for more tension. Return to start and perform eight to twelve reps.

6

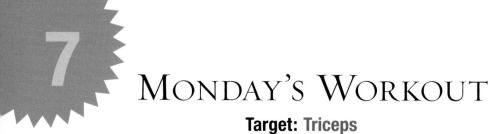

Monday's Workout
Target: Triceps

Kick Backs

- Begin exercise by standing in front of a stabilizer ball. Hold a dumbbell in your right hand.

- Bend forward and support your body by keeping the left hand on stabilizer ball. Bend your right arm ninety degrees, and keep elbows tight against the body. Remember to keep your knees slightly bent, core flexed, and head down.

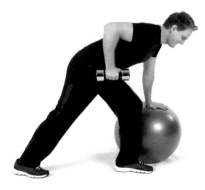

- Exhale and lift the dumbbell by extending the arm until the arm is straight and parallel to the back (If you cannot fully straighten your arm, decrease the weight until you can.)

- Hold this position for two seconds before inhaling, and slowly return your arm to a ninety-degree angle. Perform eight to twelve repetitions.

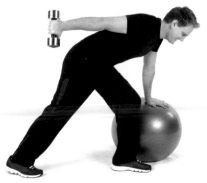

WEDNESDAY'S WORKOUT

Target: Abdominals

Toe Reach

- Lie flat on floor.

- Lift your legs straight up with knees fully extended. Point toes and raise arms in the direction of your feet.

- Exhale and slowly lift your shoulders off the ground. Reach for your toes.

- Hold for two seconds, then inhale and lower your shoulders back down to starting position.

- Do eight to twelve repetitions.

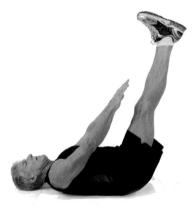
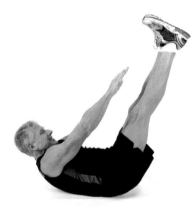

2 WEDNESDAY'S WORKOUT

Target: Core

Rotating Bird Dog

- Kneel on the floor with hands firmly placed about shoulder width apart.

- Brace the abdominals, and at first, practice lifting one hand and the opposite knee just clear of the floor while balancing on the other hand and knee. Half an inch will do until you get the idea of it.

- When you're ready to do the complete exercise, point the arm out straight in front and extend the opposite leg to the rear (see photos).

- Hold for ten seconds, and eventually work up to thirty to sixty seconds. Then return to hands and knees on ground position.

- Starting out, try five reps on alternate hands and knees—ten reps in all. Add additional sets of ten exercises up to three sets of ten.

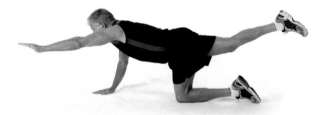

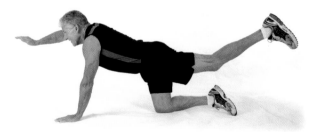

WEDNESDAY'S WORKOUT

Target: Legs

Forward Lunge With Chair

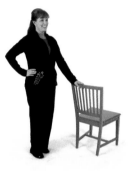

- Begin by standing next to the back portion of a sturdy chair. With your right hip facing the chair, go ahead and hold the back of the chair with your right hand for support.

- Inhale and step forward with the left foot about three feet.

- Slowly bend both knees until your right knee reaches two to three inches above the ground. Hold this position for two seconds.

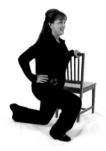

- Exhale and push through your left heel back to starting position.

- Remember to maintain good posture throughout the exercise by pulling the shoulders back, chest out, and head up.

- Perform this exercise for eight to twelve repetitions before turning around and working the right leg for eight to twelve repetitions.

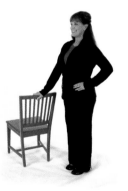

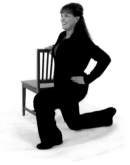

WEDNESDAY'S WORKOUT

Target: Chest

Bent Knee Push-ups

- Lie with your stomach flat against the floor. Lift feet off floor, bringing heels toward your buttocks. Bend knees to form a forty-five-degree angle or L shape. Place hands next to your body at shoulder height, keeping elbows bent.

- Exhale (breathe out through mouth) as you push your body weight off the floor by extending arms from a bent elbow to straight elbow. Be sure to have proper alignment: a straight back with ears, shoulders, and hips in a straight line. Hold abdominal muscles in tightly (pretend you are squeezing your belly button into your spine).

- Inhale (breathe in through nose) as you bend elbows and allow your body to lower to floor level. Lower your body until your face is about two to three inches from the floor.

- Repeat for a set of eight to twelve repetitions.

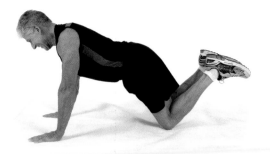

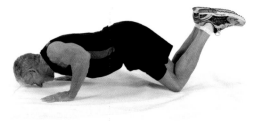

WEDNESDAY'S WORKOUT

Target: Back

Back Flies With Resistance Band

- Begin by sitting on the ground with your legs fully extended. Place the resistance band around both feet and hold on to both handles with palms facing each other, arms extended. Maintain good posture by pushing your chest out, shoulders back, head up, and flexing the core.

- Exhale and, with your elbows slightly bent, bring yours arms out to your sides. Pause when your range of motion reaches the plane of your back.

- Inhale and release back to starting position. Perform eight to twelve repetitions.

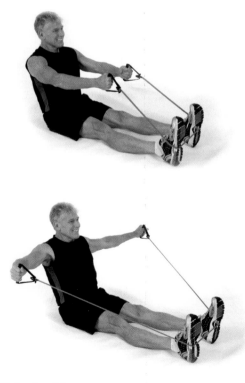

Wednesday's Workout

Target: Shoulders and Biceps

Lateral Raise (Chair or Standing) to Bicep Curl

- Begin by standing with good posture (shoulders back, head up, and chest out) with your knees slightly bent. Hang your hands down by your side with palms facing each other.

- For shoulders: Exhale and slowly raise the arms out to your sides. Bring the weight up until the point where your hands are even with your chin.

- For bicep curls: Exhale and slowly raise the arms with elbows bent. Inhale and slowly return your hands to your side.

- You may also do this exercise sitting down. Perform one repetition for shoulders, then one curl, and alternate. Perform eight to twelve reps for both shoulders and biceps.

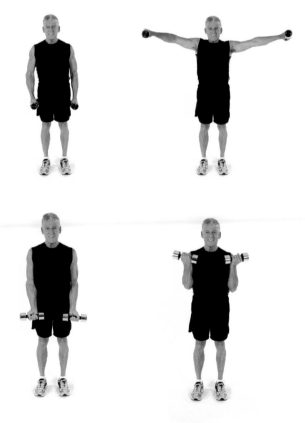

WEDNESDAY'S WORKOUT

Target: Triceps

Chair Dips

- Sit on the front edge of a sturdy chair or bench, hands close by your sides and fingers forward.

- With your legs extended, flex your feet so that your weight is on your heels.

- Feather your breathing as you slide away from the chair and bend your elbows to lower yourself until you are a few inches above the ground.

- Lift yourself back to the starting position through a count of ten seconds.

- Perform eight to twelve repetitions without resting.

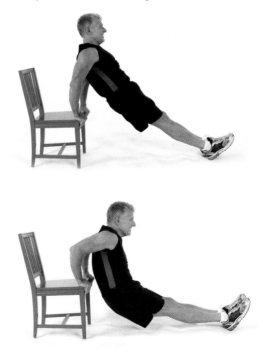

7

FRIDAY'S WORKOUT

Target: Abdominals

V Bends

- Begin exercise by sitting on the floor. Rest your hands on the floor to maintain balance throughout the exercise. Lift your legs while keeping feet together.

- Inhale and slowly lean back, extending your legs out while maintaining balance with the hands on the ground.

- Exhale and slowly bring your knees to your chest while also leaning slightly forward.

- Repeat this exercise for eight to twelve reps.

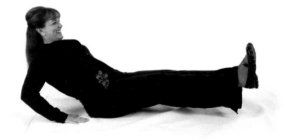

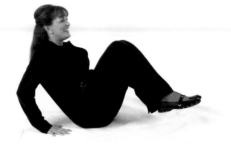

FRIDAY'S WORKOUT

Target: Abdominals

Elbows to Knees

- Lie flat on the floor, keeping your lower back and head in contact with the floor, placing your hands on the side of your head. Lift both feet off the floor, keeping your ankles and knees together throughout the movement, while keeping your lower back pulled in to the floor.

- Inhale and smoothly pull your knees toward your elbows. Avoid letting the legs come up or go out too far, as this can cause injury to the lower back.

- Squeezing a soft ball between your knees during the movement can make the exercise harder. Focus on keeping your abs contracted throughout, especially on the outward phase, where your feet should not touch the floor.

- Beginners aim for eight to twelve reps, not at full extension outward with the floor. Rest for twenty to thirty seconds, then perform again.

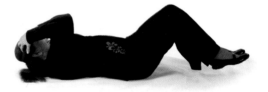

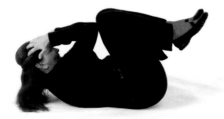

2

FRIDAY'S WORKOUT

Target: Legs

Reverse Lunge With Chair

- Begin by standing next to the back portion of a sturdy chair. With your right hip facing the chair and with your torso straight, step one foot backward about eighteen to twenty-four inches while holding the back of the chair for support.

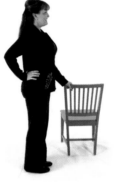
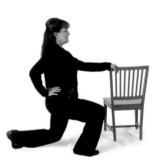

- Immediately bend the knees and descend onto the front leg, allowing the back knee to come close to the ground.

- Keep the weight on the front heel, and maintain a straight torso.

- Push back up with the back foot, and return to the standing position.

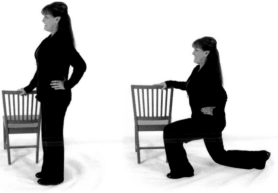

- Remember to maintain good posture throughout the exercise by pulling the shoulders back, chest out, and head up.

- Repeat this exercise for eight to twelve repetitions before turning around and working the other leg for eight to twelve reps.

FRIDAY'S WORKOUT

Target: Chest

Dumbbell Flies on Bench or Floor

- Begin by lying on your back either on a bench or the floor. Keep your hands on the side of your chest.

- Exhale through your mouth and extend your arms straight up with your palms facing each other. Then slowly inhale as you release your arms away from each other (think of a butterfly spreading its wings) and stop when your arms have made a straight line from left hand to torso to right hand (while keeping elbows slightly bent).

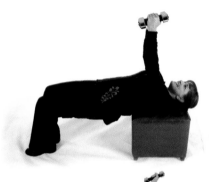

- Hold this position for two seconds, then exhale and bring your palms together while keeping your elbows slightly bent.

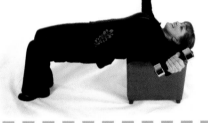

- Perform this exercise for eight to twelve repetitions while keeping your core (stomach) flexed and tight.

- OPTION: You can do this exercise with resistance bands on a bench (see photos).

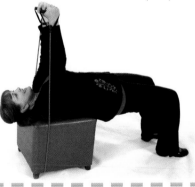

4

Friday's Workout

Target: Back

Sit-Down Band Back Flies to Back Row

- Sit on the floor with your feet together and wrap a band around your feet. Keep your knees slightly bent and the back of your heels on the floor, lean your upper body slightly forward, and maintain neutral alignment in your lower back.

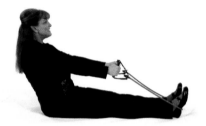

- Hold one handle in each hand. Straighten arms and position hands in front of knees with palms facing down. Tighten abdominal muscles and sit upright with shoulders back.

- Begin with hands together and palms facing each other. Keep arms extended with elbows slightly bent. Exhale through your mouth as your bring your arms apart until your left hand, torso, and right hand all make a straight line. Then inhale through your nose as you release your hands to the starting position with palms facing each other.

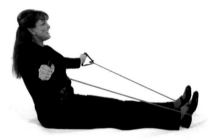

- Keep the wrists firm and unbent. Slowly bend the arms and pull elbows straight back while keeping elbows tight against the side. Pull your elbows past your hips, hold one to two seconds, and slowly return to start position.

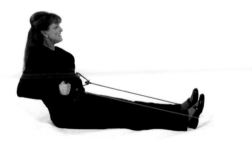

- Inhale and release the hands back to the starting position.

- Do each movement for eight to twelve repetitions.

FRIDAY'S WORKOUT

Target: Shoulders and Arms

Hammer Frontal Raise to Hammer Curl

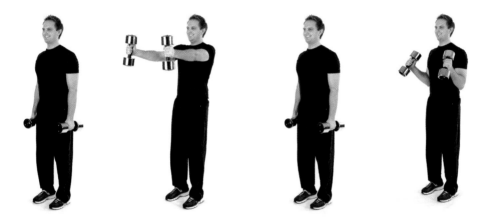

- Begin by standing with your feet shoulder width apart. Keep weights by your side with palms facing each other. Maintain good posture, shoulders back, head back, chest out, and core tight.

- Exhale and bring the weights up to chin level while keeping arms fully extended.

- Inhale and slowly release to starting position with hands by side.

- Exhale again and keep palms facing each other as you curl the arms in until the weights tap the bicep.

- Inhale and slowly lower the weights back to starting position.

- Alternate each exercise for eight to twelve repetitions (eight to twelve frontal raises and eight to twelve hammer curls).

6

FRIDAY'S WORKOUT

Target: Triceps

Door Pull-downs on Bands

- Begin by opening up any stable door to a forty-five-degree angle and placing the middle of the band over the top portion of the door.

- Grab both handles and step about six inches away from the door.

- Take a neutral position (feet shoulder width apart with one foot slightly in front of the other with legs slightly bent). Keep your elbows tight to your side and palms facing the ground with your elbows bent to a ninety-degree angle.

- Exhale and bring your arms down until they are fully extended. Hold this position for two seconds, inhale, and slowly release until your elbows are back to a ninety-degree position.

- Perform this exercise for eight to twelve repetitions.

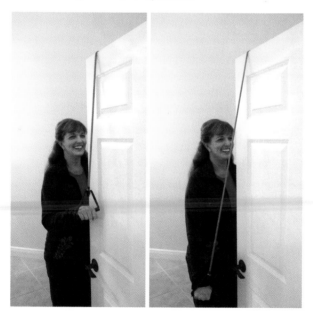

Benefits of Rebounding

Albert E. Carter, author of *Rebound Exercise: The Ultimate Exercise for the New Millennium*, has experienced firsthand the various health benefits of rebounding throughout his life. He can perform 100 hundred push-ups and has never lifted weights in his life. He taught both of his children to rebound from a very early age. His son, Daren, was able to do 429 sit-ups the first time he was challenged (in the first grade) and his daughter, Wendy, was able to do 476 sit-ups without stopping and beat all the boys in her sixth grade class in arm wrestling even though she had never arm wrestled before! It's interesting that the only exercise they did was to jump on a trampoline.

In addition to strengthening your muscles, rebounding is becoming more recognized for its benefits in fighting cancer due to the way it helps improve your body's lymphatic flow. For more information on rebounding, refer to page 164–165.

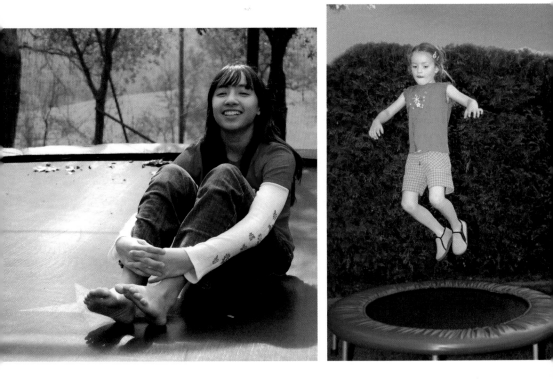

9

THE GET FIT AND LIVE WORKOUT FOR INTERMEDIATE AND ADVANCED

Important!

Before undergoing any activity or fitness program, please check with your doctor to make sure that you are healthy enough to participate.

IN THIS CHAPTER, WE'VE created three intermediate workouts and three advanced workouts. As with the beginner workouts in chapter 8, the plan is to give you a workout consisting of seven exercises that you can complete in seven minutes every Monday, Wednesday, and Friday. So when you turn the page, you'll see instructions and photos for the first two exercises for Monday's workout. As the chapter progresses you'll learn how to do all seven exercises for Monday, Wednesday, and Friday.

Here are a few tips to help you make the most of your workout:

- **Timing:** To complete these workouts in seven minutes, your goal should be to perform each exercise for thirty seconds, and then rebound (jump on a minitrampoline) for thirty seconds before moving on to the next exercise. (For instructions on rebounding, see pages 164–165.)

- **Before and after:** We recommend that you warm up with the seven-minute rebounding routinein chapter 16 before your workout, and that you cool down with stretches we've provided for you in chapter 10.

- **Equipment:** For these workouts you'll need some light to medium dumbbells, a resistance band, a bosu, a stabilizer ball, and Perfect Pushups (optional). You'll also need a rebounder for the warm up and thirty-second intervals between exercises.

- **Household items:** You'll need a sturdy chair and an ottoman or bench.

- **Progression:** As you become better conditioned, you may increase your number of sets per exercise to two or three sets. You may also increase the intensity of our workouts by slowing increasing your weights; however, keep your repetitions consistent.

If you're starting out with these intermediate workouts, you may have skipped chapter 8 where we reminded you that as a bonus for purchasing this book, we've made the videotaped demonstrations of several stretches and exercises we produced for *The Seven Pillars of Health* available to you. If you'd like to download this FREE twenty-minute video, visit www.sevenpillarsofhealth.com. NOTE: The video is not required for the workouts we're about to explain. It's additional coaching and instruction above and beyond what we've provided in this book. Some of the exercises and stretches in the video are the same as what you'll find on these pages, and some are different.

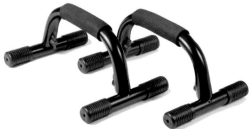

If you skipped chapter 8, we encourage you to turn back to the opening page for just a moment and read the "Dr. Colbert Approved" way to breathe during your workout. If you have any health conditions, check with your doctor before working out and read the remaining chapters in this book where we've explained how to customize these workouts for people with diabetes, osteoporosis, arthritis, chronic fatigue, fibromyalgia, and more.

As you regularly perform these workouts, your fitness will increase. After a few months you may be ready to move from the intermediate to the advanced workouts. But this isn't a race, so take your time. Some people will never be able to progress to the intermediate or advanced level, and that's perfectly fine. The goal is to be healthy and keep your body moving. It's time to get fit and live! Are you ready? Turn the page and let's get started!

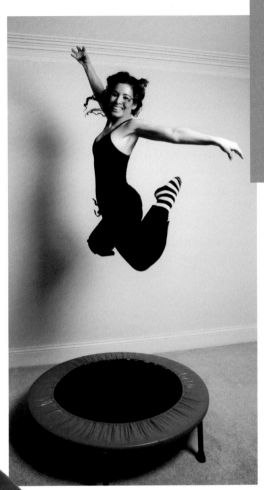

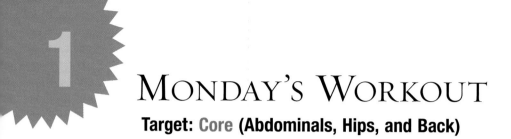

Monday's Workout

Target: Core (Abdominals, Hips, and Back)

Intermediate: Pique on Stabilizer Ball

- Start off on the ball in push-up position with your shin stabilized on the ball.

- Note: If you have trouble getting into starting position, start with your stomach on the ball and slowly roll yourself forward with your hands walking you to push-up position.

- Keep your abs flexed, and inhale through your nose as you pull your knees to your chest.

- Exhale through your mouth and straighten your legs back to push-up position.

- Maintain this position for thirty to sixty seconds.

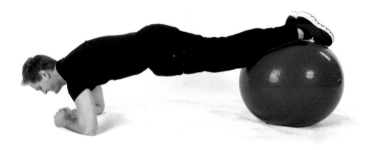

Advanced Option

- The further you roll out, the more difficult the exercise becomes. As your core gets stronger, move the ball to your toes for more resistance.

- Maintain this position for sixty to one hundred twenty seconds.

MONDAY'S WORKOUT
Target: Core (Abdominals, Hips, and Back)

Intermediate: Side Plank

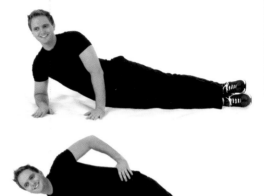

- Start off by lying on your side. Lift your torso off the ground and balance yourself on your forearm and the side of your foot.

- Contract your abdominals by flexing or sucking in your stomach.

- Remember to relax your shoulders and slowly breathe in through the nose and out through the mouth.

- Hold this position for thirty to sixty seconds.

Advanced: Side Plank on Stabilizer Ball

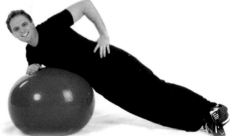

- Start off by balancing yourself on your forearm and side on a stabilizer ball.

- Contract your abdominals by flexing or sucking in your stomach as you lift your torso off of the ball.

- Remember to relax your shoulders and slowly breathe in through the nose and out through the mouth.

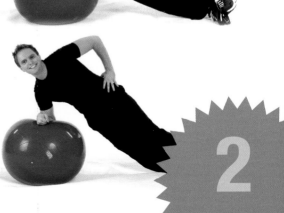

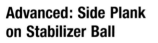

2

MONDAY'S WORKOUT

Target: Legs and Biceps

Intermediate: Chair Squat to Shoulder Press

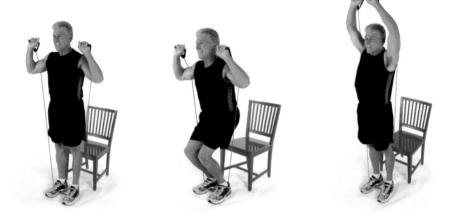

- Start off by standing two to four inches away from a chair with your back facing the chair. Stand with your feet shoulder width apart while anchoring the tubing under both feet.

- Continue holding the bands at shoulder height while keeping your palms facing out. Inhale through your nose as you bend your knees while keeping your shoulders and neck back. Hover yourself one to two inches above the chair for two seconds, then stand up straight while keeping knees slightly bent at standing position.

- At standing position exhale through the mouth as you raise arms above the head and fully extend arms and elbows. Inhale through the nose and release your hands back down to the shoulders.

- Perform chair squat to shoulder press for eight to twelve reps.

Target: Legs and Shoulders

Advanced: Ball Squat to Shoulder Press

- Begin by placing the ball on the lower part of the back. Hold the weights up by your shoulders. Maintain good posture: shoulders back, head back, and core tight.

- Inhale and slowly bend your knees until your legs make a 90-degree angle. Hold for two seconds.

- Exhale and extend your legs (never fully straighten the knee).

- Then bring the weights up above your head.

- Straighten your elbows until the weights touch. Hold for two seconds, and then slowly release your elbows back down to your shoulder.

- Do eight to twelve repetitions.

MONDAY'S WORKOUT

Target: Chest and Triceps

Intermediate: Chest Press on Stabilizer Ball to Tricep Extension

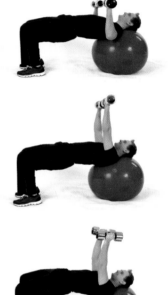

- Start off so that the ball is resting comfortably in the center of your back. Roll downward until the ball supports your head. Lift up your torso so that the area from your chest to your knees makes a straight line.

- Position your elbows to the side with your palms facing in the direction of your feet. Exhale through your mouth and extend your arms up so that the weights barely touch each other.

- As your arms are extended, face your palms toward each other and bend your elbows so that the weight will slowly move past your ears. Make a ninety-degree angle with your arms and hold for two seconds before exhaling through your mouth and extending your elbows, bringing your weights straight up.

- Turn your palms to face toward your feet. Inhale through your nose and release your arms again so that the weights go back to your sides.

- Intermediates should perform this exercise for eight to twelve reps.

Advanced Option

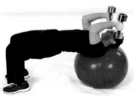

- As you become more comfortable on the ball and continue to strengthen your muscles, try increasing the weight by five pounds every few weeks. Also, bring your feet closer together, which requires more stability.

MONDAY'S WORKOUT

Target: Back

Intermediate: Arm Haulers

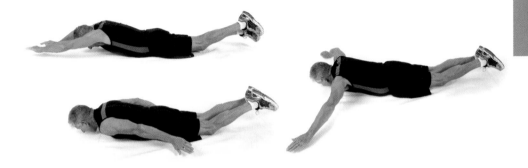

- Begin by laying flat on your stomach with feet a few inches off the floor. Keep your arms extended above your head with your hands touching. Position your head facing down toward the ground to maintain good alignment of your neck and spine.

- Slowly bring your arms around to your side while keeping your arms fully extended. (Think of doing a snow angel without moving your feet.) Remember not to hold your breath, but instead slowly feather your breathing as you bring your arms together over your head and back down to your sides.

- Perform this exercise for twenty seconds or eight to twelve repetitions (one repetition equals bringing your hands down to your sides and back together over your head).

Advanced Option

- Try holding 2½- or 5-pound dumbbells while doing this exercise.

- Do eight to twelve reps without letting the weights touch the floor.

Monday's Workout
Target: Lower Back

Intermediate: Back Extension on Bosu

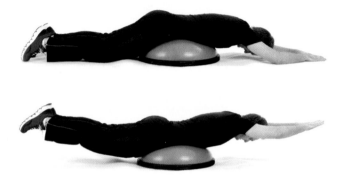

- Begin by lying down facedown on the bosu with your belly button over the center of the bubble.

- Bring hands together and extend them straight out over your head.

- Maintain a flexed stomach while you left your feet, head, and arms off the ground.

- Hold this position for ten seconds, then repeat for eight to twelve repetitions.

Advanced Option:

- Try holding 2½- to 5-pound dumbbells and/or wear 2½- to 5-pound ankle weights.

- Hold the position for three to five seconds between reps, and increase the reps to twelve to fifteen.

MONDAY'S WORKOUT
Target: Shoulders

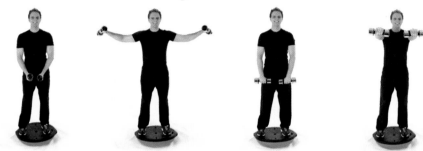

Intermediate: Frontal Raise to Lateral Raise on Bosu

- Begin by balancing your feet on the flat side of the bosu. Remember, the goal is to remain as steady on the bosu as possible. While maintaining balance, hold the weights together in front of you with your palms facing each other. Maintain good posture by keeping your feet shoulder width apart, knees slightly bent, elbows slightly bent, chest out, shoulders back, and head up.

- Exhale and bring the weights out and up to your side while keeping the elbow slightly bent. Bring the weights up until your right arm, shoulders, and left arm make a straight line (think of making a cross).

- Hold this position for two seconds, inhale, and release the weights back down to starting position. Keep your elbows slightly bent, exhale, and rotate your hands in so that your palms are facing the floor, bring the weights straight up in front of you until it reaches the height of your chin.

- Hold this position for two seconds, inhale, and release the weights back down to your side. Then perform the lateral raise again.

- Intermediate should repeat until you have completed eight to twelve frontal raises and eight to twelve lateral raises.

Advanced Option

- You should gradually increase weight every few weeks. Also, try holding the weight longer at the apex of your exercise. For example, when you lift your arms up on the lateral raise and frontal raise, try holding that position for five seconds. This helps fatigue the muscle, which allows you to avoid any plateaus.

- TIP: Remember, the key to this exercise is slow, controlled movements.

7

Wednesday's Workout

Target: Abdominals

Intermediate/Advanced: Ball Pass

- Begin by lying on your back with the legs and arms straight up while holding the stabilizer ball between the legs and hands.

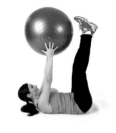

- Release your hands and let the feet hold on to the ball by squeezing with the thighs.

- Lower both arms and legs at the same time toward the floor.

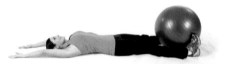

- Then bring the feet and hands up and exchange the ball from the legs to the hands.

- Again, bring your hands and feet back down to the ground while holding on to the ball.

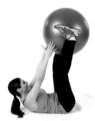

- Intermediate should perform this exercise for fifteen to twenty repetitions.

- Advanced should perform this exercise for twenty to thirty repetitions or more.

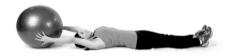

WEDNESDAY'S WORKOUT

Target: Abs and Core

Intermediate: Plank on Bosu

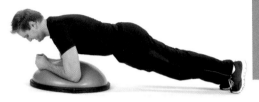

- Begin by laying facedown with your forearms and palms resting on the bosu.

- Push off the bosu, rising up onto your toes, and remain resting on the elbows. The key is to keep your back as flat as possible from head to heels.

- Slightly tilt your pelvis in and contract or squeeze your abdominals, which will keep your rear from sticking too high in the air.

- Hold this position for thirty to sixty seconds.

Advanced: Plank on Bosu With Leg Lifts

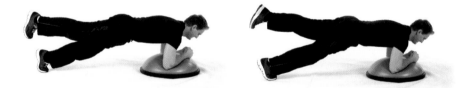

- Begin by laying facedown with your forearms and palms resting on bosu.

- Push off the bosu, rising up onto your toes, and remain resting on the elbows. The key is to keep your back as flat as possible from head to heels.

- Slightly tilt your pelvis in and contract or squeeze your abdominals, which will keep your rear from sticking too high in the air. Lift your right leg.

- Hold this position for thirty to sixty seconds. Return leg to the floor.

- Repeat ten to twelve times for right leg. Then switch legs for ten to twelve more reps.

2

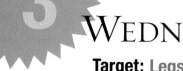

WEDNESDAY'S WORKOUT

Target: Legs and Shoulders

Intermediate: Ball Squat to Front Raises

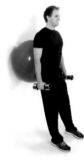

- Begin by placing the ball on the lower part of the back. Use a sturdy wall to stabilize the ball behind you. Lean back on the ball and walk out one and a half to two feet. Hold the weights up by your shoulders with your palms facing away from you.

- Inhale, and slowly bend your knees until your knees reach a ninety-degree angle. (Note: If your knees go past the plane of your toes, you need to walk out further.)

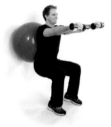

- Exhale and extend the legs. Remember never to lock the knees but to keep them slightly bent.

- Exhale again, and slowly bring the weights to chin height with your arms fully extended and the weights touching.

- Inhale and slowly bring the weights back down.

- Perform this combination exercise for ten to twelve repetitions.

Target: Back, Buttocks, and Hamstrings

Advanced: T-Back Fly

- Begin by holding weights by your side.

- Exhale and slowly lean forward while at the same time bringing the weights out to your side. Also lift the right leg straight back so that both arms and right leg are parallel to the floor.

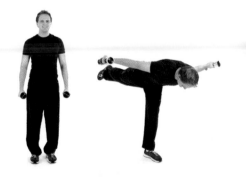

- Pause once your arms and right leg make a T.

- Inhale and slowly return to starting position.

- Repeat the exercise on the other leg. Continue rotating legs until you reach twenty-four reps (twelve on the right leg and twelve on the left leg).

WEDNESDAY'S WORKOUT

Target: Chest

Intermediate: Push-ups With Legs on Stabilizer Ball

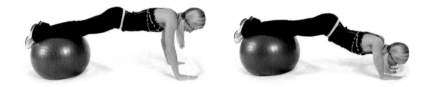

- Get into push-up position with your feet on the stabilizer ball. Keep your legs straight.

- Exhale, and push your body up until your arms are almost fully extended. (Do not lock your elbows.) Hold this position for two to three seconds.

- Inhale, and slowly lower yourself until your chest grazes the floor.

- Perform fifteen to twenty repetitions.

Advanced: Push-ups on Stabilizer Ball

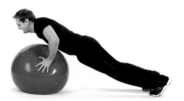

- Begin by laying your chest on the stabilizer ball. Place your hands by the sides of your chest. Keep your toes on the floor while keeping your legs straight.

- Exhale, and push your body up until your arms are almost fully extended. (Do not lock your elbows.) Hold this position for two to three seconds.

- Inhale, and slowly lower yourself until your chest grazes the ball.

- Perform fifteen to twenty repetitions.

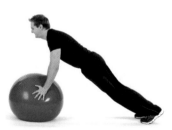

WEDNESDAY'S WORKOUT

Target: Back

Intermediate/Advanced:
Upper Back Row to Lower
Back Row on Stabilizer Ball

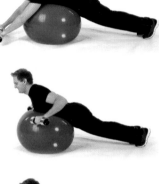

- Begin by laying facedown on the ball with the ball resting underneath your belly button. Stretch out your legs so that only your toes are maintaining your balance on the ball. Make sure to keep your chest out and shoulders back, while staring straight ahead.

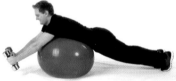

- Position your hands straight out fully extended without touching the stabilizer ball. Keep your palms facing each other, exhale, and pull your elbows back until your elbow touches your side. Hold that position for two seconds, inhale, and release back to starting position.

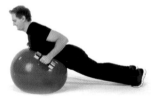

- Complete eight to twelve reps. Turn dumbbells to vertical position and perform eight to twelve reps.

(Alternate view)

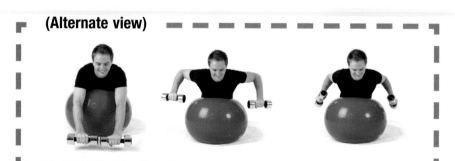

WEDNESDAY'S WORKOUT

Target: Shoulders and Biceps

Intermediate: Shoulder Press on Bosu

- Begin by standing on the flat side of the bosu. Keep your feet shoulder width apart, shoulders back, head up, and chest out. Hold the weights.

- Exhale and lift the weights slowly over your head until your arms and shoulders make a straight line.

- Hold this position for two seconds, inhale, and slowly release back to starting position.

- Intermediates should perform eight to twelve repetitions.

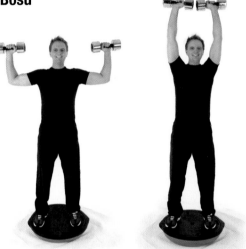

Advanced Option

- Perform eight to twelve reps, but hold the arms up position for five seconds. Increase weights by five pounds every few weeks as able.

WEDNESDAY'S WORKOUT

Target: Triceps

Intermediate/Advanced: Close Grip Push-ups on Bosu

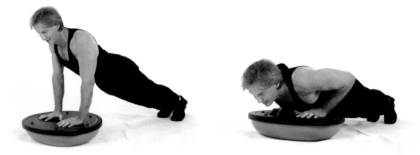

- Begin by placing your palms on the flat side of the bosu with your thumbs touching each other.

- Extend your legs back so that only your toes are touching the floor and your body is straight.

- Inhale and bend your elbows slightly to tense up your tricep muscles.

- Keeping your body straight, slowly lower your body until your nose is one inch from the bosu. Hold this position for two seconds.

- Exhale and push back up to the starting position without locking your elbows.

- Intermediates, perform this exercise for eight to twelve slow reps.

Advanced Option

- Try the extra challenge of doing these push-ups with your feet elevated on a step or bench.

FRIDAY'S WORKOUT

Target: Abdominals

Intermediate: V Bends

- Begin exercise by sitting on the floor. Keep your hands by your sides, not on the floor. Extend your legs out while keeping feet together.

- Slowly lean back and lift feet off the ground while maintaining balance.

- Exhale, and slowly bring your knees to your chest while also leaning slightly forward.

- Inhale and lean back while at the same time extending your legs to starting position.

- Repeat for fifteen to twenty repetitions.

Advanced: V Bends on Bosu

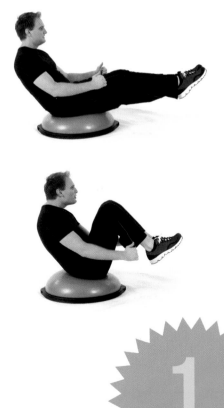

- Begin exercise by sitting on the bosu. Rest your hands on the sides of the bosu to maintain balance throughout the exercise.

- Extend your legs out while keeping feet together. Slowly lean back and lift feet off the ground while maintaining balance with the hands on the bosu.

- Exhale and slowly bring your knees to your chest while also leaning slightly forward.

- Inhale and lean back while at the same time extending your legs back to the starting position.

- Repeat this exercise for twenty or more reps.

1

2

FRIDAY'S WORKOUT

Target: Core (Abdominals, Lower Back, and Hips)

Intermediate: Ball Circles

- Place your forearms on a stabilizer ball, and extend your legs behind you at hip width apart.

- Flex your core and raise yourself into a plank position. Using your forearms, roll the ball out to the left, in front of you, and back to the right (think of a stirring motion).

- This is one repetition. Perform this exercise for eight to twelve repetitions.

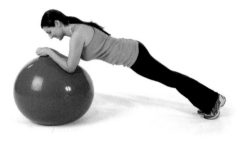

Advanced: Ball Plank With Leg Lift

- Get into plank position with the arms resting on the ball.

- Make sure your hands are under your shoulders with your abs contracted.

- Lift the right leg off the floor a few inches and lower and perform on the other leg.

- Alternate legs for fifteen reps.

- TIP: Prop the ball against the wall for balance.

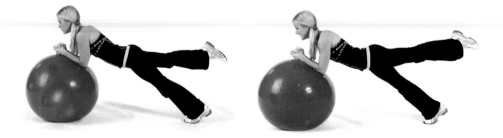

FRIDAY'S WORKOUT
Target: Legs

Intermediate: One-Legged Lunge With Chair or Bench

- Begin by placing the left foot/shin on bench or chair.

- Step out so that your right leg is two to three feet away from the chair.

- Inhale and slowly bend your knee until it reaches a 90-degree angle.

- Hold this position for several seconds.

- Exhale and slow extend knee back to starting position.

- Do eight to twelve reps for each leg.

- TIP: Place hands on hips for better stability.

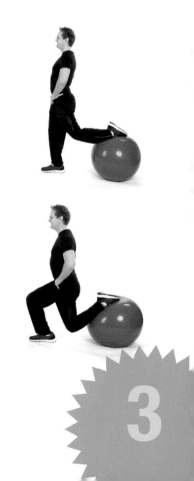

Advanced: One-Legged Lunge

- Begin by placing the left foot/shin on the ball.

- Bend the right knee into a lunge position as you roll the ball out with your left leg.

- Inhale and slowly bend the right knee to a ninety-degree angle while making sure the knee stays behind the toe.

- Exhale and push through the right heel until the leg is almost straight. (Note: never fully extend the leg and always keep slightly bent.)

- After ten to twelve repetitions, switch legs for ten to twelve more repetitions.

- TIP: This exercise requires balance, so you might need to use a wall for balance when positioning yourself on the ball.

3

FRIDAY'S WORKOUT

Target: Chest

Intermediate/Advanced: Ball Chest Fly to Pullover

- Begin by lying back on the stabilizer ball with your shoulders and neck resting on the majority of the ball. Keep your feet shoulder width apart, and raise your rear so that your torso makes a straight line. Hold two weights in your hand with palms facing toward your toes.

- Exhale and extend your arms up until the weights touch.

- Inhale, keeping your arms extended, and slowly bring the weights over your head until your hands are directly behind your head.

- Exhale and bring the weights back above your chest.

- Inhale and slowly release the weights back to the starting position.

- Perform this exercise for eight to twelve repetitions of chest flies and eight to twelve pullovers.

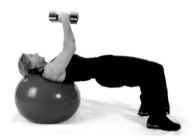
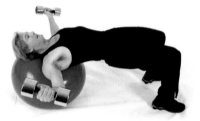
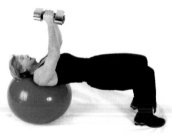
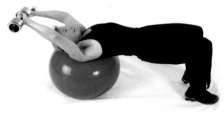

FRIDAY'S WORKOUT

Target: Triceps and Chest

Intermediate: Perfect Push-ups on Stabilizer Ball

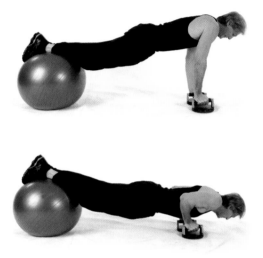

- Begin by getting into push-up position with your feet and lower legs resting on the ball. You can either place your palms flat on the floor or grip two Perfect Pushup units (as shown).

- Inhale and bend your elbows slightly to tense up your tricep muscles.

- Keeping your body straight, slowly lower your body until your nose is one inch from the floor. Hold this position for two seconds.

- Exhale and push back up to the starting position without locking your elbows.

- Perform this exercise for eight to twelve slow reps.

Advanced Option

- Perform twelve reps.

5

FRIDAY'S WORKOUT

Target: Shoulders and Arms

Intermediate: Arm Curls on Bosu

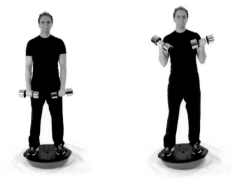

- Begin by standing on the flat side of the bosu with your feet shoulder width apart. Slightly bend your knees and hold the weights by your side. Make sure that your palms are facing each other.

- Exhale and slowly lift your left arm. As you bring up the left arm, rotate your wrist outward so that your palm is facing your body.

- Inhale and slowly release the weight back down by your side. (Remember to rotate your wrist inward so that your palm is facing your side.)

- Perform eight to twelve repetitions, and repeat with right arm for eight to twelve more reps.

Advanced: Truck Driver on Bosu

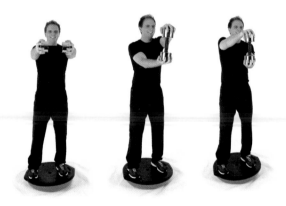

- Begin by standing on the flat side of the bosu with your feet shoulder width apart. Hold a dumbbell with both hands straight out in front of your body. Tighten your core and maintain balance while you slowly turn the weight as if you are driving a truck.

- First turn it to your left and then turn it to your right. (That is one repetition.) Maintain breathing throughout the exercise.

- Perform this exercise for eight to twelve repetitions.

FRIDAY'S WORKOUT

Target: Triceps

Intermediate: Ball Dips

- Sit on the ball and place your hands on the ball close to your hips.

- Bring the hips up and away from the ball as you straighten your arms.

- Maintain balance as you inhale through your nose and bend your arms, lowering your body back down to the ball.

- Exhale through your mouth as you extend and straighten your arm back to starting position.

- Perform for eight to twelve repetitions.

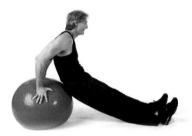

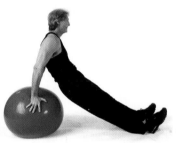

Advanced: Ball Dips on Bench

- Sit on the ball, and place your hands on the ball close to your hips. Place your feet on an ottoman or bench.

- Bring the hips up and away from the ball as you straighten your arms.

- Maintain balance as you inhale through your nose and bend your arms to form a ninety-degree angle.

- Exhale through your mouth as you extend and straighten your arm back to starting position.

- Perform for eight to twelve repetitions or more.

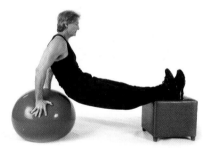

7

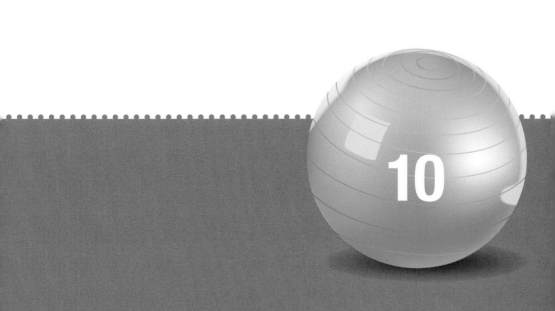

COOL DOWN WITH STRETCHES

Total Body Stretch

- Begin by sitting on the floor and extending your legs in front of you.

- Take a deep breath and then exhale and slowly reach for your ankles or toes.

- You have reached your maximum flexibility when you feel a slight discomfort in your hamstrings.

- Hold for five to ten seconds and slowly release

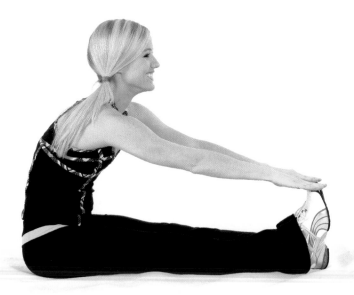

SPINAL ROTATION STRETCH

- Lie on your back with arms outstretched at shoulder level.

- Slowly drop your knees to the right until the right knee is touching the floor.

- While dropping your knees, keep your shoulder blades flat on the floor. (Note: do not force the stretch.)

- Hold this position for eight to ten seconds, and repeat with the other side.

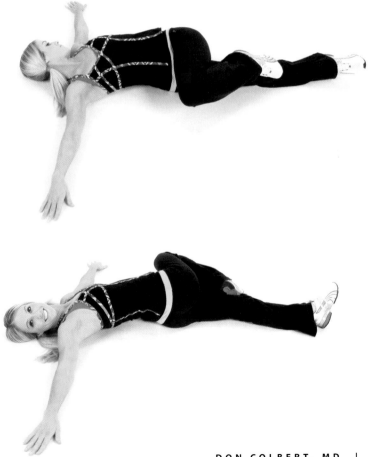

LYING KNEES TO CHEST

- Lie on the floor with your legs extended. Bend your knees in toward your chest, and separate your knees from each other. (Note: point your feet and keep your toes together.)

- Then draw your knees together, and wrap your arms around your legs.

- Roll to your right. Roll to your left.

- Perform this stretch several times.

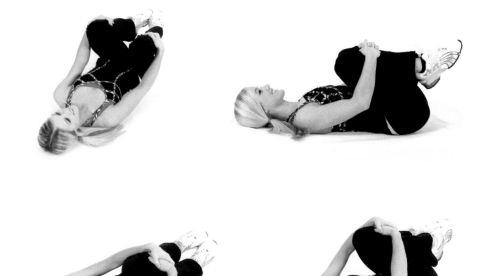

LYING PELVIC TILTS

- On a carpeted floor or stretching mat, lie on your back with your knees bent and your feet flat on the floor.

- Inhale deeply, and as you exhale, tip your pelvis upward so that you feel your lower back gently pressing against the floor. (Note: keep your upper body relaxed and free of tension. Focus on just your pelvis.)

- Release back to neutral spine position and perform eight to twelve times. (Remember to keep your upper back on the floor and your neck and shoulders relaxed.)

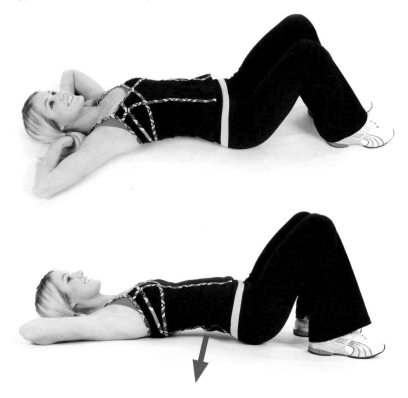

LENGTHENING BACK EXTENSION

- Begin by lying on your stomach, and bring your palms back until your lower arms are perpendicular to the floor.

- Take a deep breath, and slowly exhale as you straighten your arms, lifting your shoulders away from the ground.

- NOTE: Pull your shoulder blades together for maximum stretch.

- Hold this position for five to ten seconds.

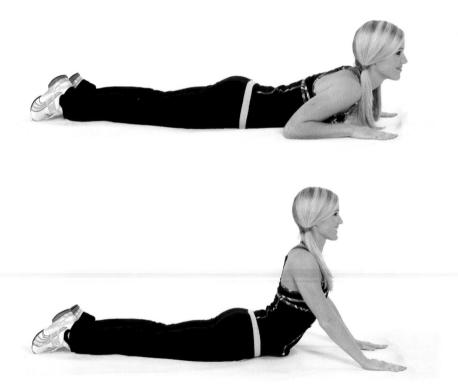

CAT POSE

- Get on the floor on your hands and knees with your hands directly under your shoulders and your knees directly under your hips. Lay the tops of your feet on the floor and point your toes back.

- Inhale and arch your back, lifting your tailbone toward the ceiling. Hold the stretch for five to ten seconds, release the position back to neutral spine, and then inhale again.

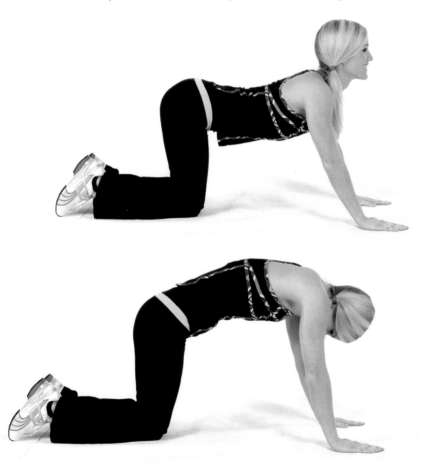

LAT STRETCH ON ALL FOURS

- Begin with your knees and your hands on the floor.

- Exhale and reach your arms straight forward and lower your chest toward the floor, keeping your hips higher than your shoulders.

- Feather your breathing, and move your shoulders and arms toward the right as far as you can reach while keeping your hips pulled to the ground.

- Hold this position for thirty seconds. Try to take four to five deep breaths throughout the stretch. (Note: you should feel a slight arch in the back and progress through this stretch gradually.)

- Repeat, moving shoulders and arms toward the left.

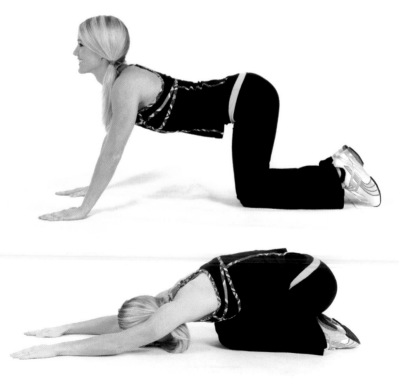

BUTTOCKS STRETCH

- While lying on your back, cross the right leg over the left knee.

- Grab the left leg with both hands around the back of the thigh, and press the elbow into the right knee.

- Gradually pull back with both hands as you press forward with the elbow.

- Hold for twenty to thirty seconds.

- Repeat for other leg.

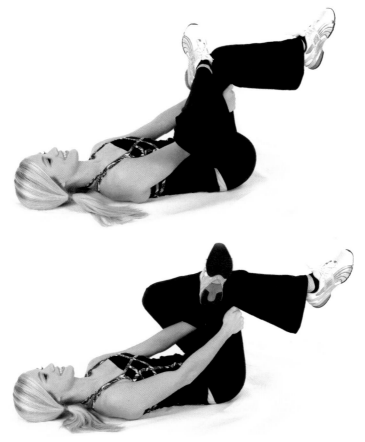

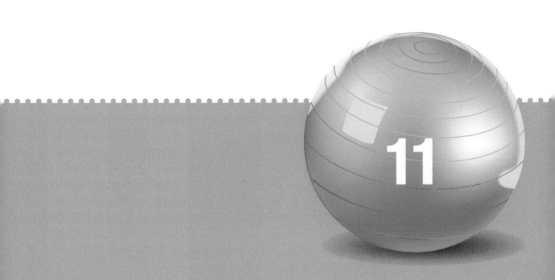

TARGETING WEIGHT LOSS

EXERCISE: *THE* WEIGHT-LOSS SUPPLEMENT

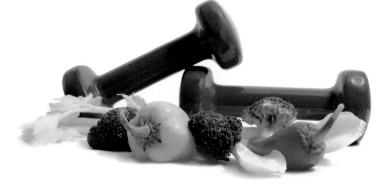

THERE IS NO BETTER way to complement a diet or weight-loss eating program than by being physically active on a regular basis. How does exercise specifically help with losing weight? The ways are just as plentiful as the overall benefits of exercise. First, regular physical activity helps raise the metabolic rate both during exercise and for hours afterward. It also enables you to develop more muscle, which raises the metabolic rate all day long and even while you're sleeping. Daily exercise decreases body fat and improves your ability to cope with stress by lowering the stress hormone cortisol (which is a major cause of fat).

Such activity also raises serotonin levels, which helps to reduce cravings for sweets and carbohydrates. It assists in burning off dangerous belly fat and improves your body's ability to handle sugar. Finally, exercising on a regular basis can even help control your appetite by boosting serotonin levels, lowering cortisol, and decreasing insulin levels (which can also decrease your chances for insulin resistance).

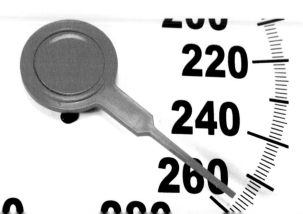

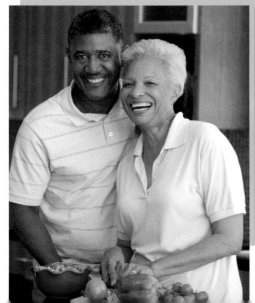

Dr. Colbert Approved

Basic Workout for Losing Weight

If weight loss is your goal, I recommend using the workout in chapter 7 of this book for one to two months or until you can perform the exercises fairly easily. Then you can adapt the workout as follows to really start targeting weight loss as your goal. (For more details on targeting your workout for weight loss, refer to *Dr. Colbert's "I Can Do This" Diet*.)

- Start with a five- to ten-minute warm-up on the treadmill or rebounder at low intensity but in your fat-burning zone. The fat-burning zone is the lower end of your target heart rate zone, or around 65–70 percent of your predicted maximum heart rate. (The target heart rate zone is 65–85 percent, but the fat-burning zone is usually around 65–70 percent.)

- Second, I recommend about fifteen to thirty minutes of calisthenics, weight training, or resistance band exercises at least three times a week (every other day). The resistance exercises help to deplete the glycogen stores (or stored sugar) from the liver and muscles. The beginner workout in chapter 8 is for only seven minutes, but eventually, by increasing sets, it will be fifteen to thirty minutes.

- Third, I recommend approximately twenty to thirty minutes of aerobic exercise in the fat-burning zone. (See the formula on page 33 to figure out your target heart rate.) Staying at 65–75 percent of your maximum heart rate is your fat-burning zone.

- Last, I recommend a five- to ten-minute cooldown. I usually have my patients end with the stretches I provided for you in chapter 10.

Hitting a Plateau

If you lose weight steadily and then seem to hit a plateau, exercise can help. Some people find that increasing the frequency and duration of exercise helps them break through a plateau and resume losing weight. If you don't exercise at all, you need to start! If you already exercise, try to increase your exercise time gradually. Each week, add five additional minutes of exercise per day until you reach forty-five minutes a day.

Power Cardio Workouts

HIGH-INTENSITY ANAEROBIC WORKOUTS OBVIOUSLY have proven value. Not only that, but studies in recent years have shown that these "power cardio" routines can be just as effective as longer, moderate-intensity workouts. It's no surprise, then, that the American public, with its usual "faster is better" mind-set, has adopted this as the preferred way to lose fat. However, after helping thousands of overweight and obese individuals successfully lose weight and keep it off, we believe we have enough credentials to speak on this matter. And to us, it comes down to staying the course.

Remember all the diets you've tried in the past? Remember all the New Year's Days you committed to joining the gym and working out more? What happened in each of these cases? Your commitment fizzled. Something got in the way and distracted you enough to veer you from your ultimate goal. It's the same way with being active. I believe the biggest obstacle for most obese individuals is not working out; it's adopting that activity as part of a lifestyle.

Let us offer a suggestion for those who have exercised religiously in the past or who are quickly bored with moderate-intensity workouts. Try varying it up once in a while with some high-intensity interval training (HIIT). Notice the word *interval*, however. This is simply alternating between brief, hard bursts of exercise and short stretches of lower-intensity exercise or rest. Various studies in recent years have proven this to be an effective way to improve not only overall cardiovascular health but also your ability to burn fat faster. One study at the University of Guelph in Ontario, Canada, found that following an interval training session with an hour of moderate cycling increased the amount of fat burned by 36 percent.[1]

Our suggestion is to hold off on HIIT, regardless of your exercise past, until you've consistently done some moderate-intensity activity for several months. We'd rather see you be able to sustain your momentum for the long haul rather than have you burn out, not because of eating the wrong things, but simply because you wanted to sprint to the finish line faster.

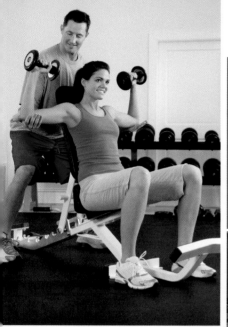

Don't Work Out Hungry

Before exercising, make sure that you have either eaten a meal two or three hours prior, or you have a healthy snack about thirty minutes to an hour before exercising. It is never good to exercise when you are hungry because you may end up burning muscle protein as energy—which is very expensive fuel since losing muscle lowers your metabolic rate.

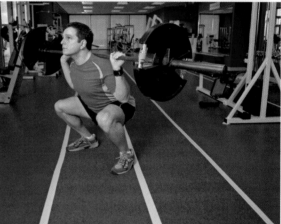

High-Intensity Interval Training (HIIT)

High-intensity interval training (HIIT) mixes high-intensity bursts of exercise with moderate-intensity recovery periods, usually for a period of less than twenty minutes. It is used mostly for individuals trying to lose weight. For more information on HIIT, see Dr. Colbert's "I Can Do This" Diet.

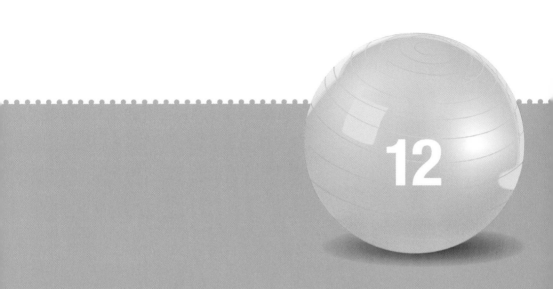

TARGETING TYPE
2 DIABETES

TARGETING TYPE 2 DIABETES

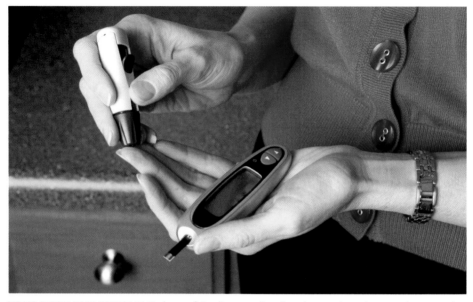

YOUR BODY, THE DWELLING place of God's Spirit, needs to be protected and kept healthy. You must take courage and continually battle diabetes because it can weaken and damage other organs in your body.

I cannot stress enough how important it is to overcome your diabetes with exercise. Exercise holds special benefits for diabetics. Multiple studies have shown that those who have a physically active lifestyle are less prone to develop type 2 diabetes. I believe this is because physical exercise battles the root of type 2 diabetes, which gets its start when muscle cells lose their sensitivity to insulin. Research has shown that your muscle cells are much less likely to resist insulin if you keep them fit through regular exercise.[1]

Studies have also shown that regular exercise improves glucose tolerance and lowers blood sugar as well as insulin requirements.[2] By helping muscles to take glucose from the bloodstream and use it for energy, exercise prevents sugar from accumulating in the blood. Also, by burning calories, exercise helps control weight, an important factor in the management of type 2 diabetes.

A study at the Cooper Institute for Aerobics Research in Dallas shows that staying fit may be the most important thing you can do to avoid type 2 diabetes. The researchers put 8,633 men with an average age of forty-three through a treadmill test and then screened them for diabetes six years later. The men who scored poorly on the fitness test were almost four times more likely to have developed the disease than those who had done well on the treadmill. In fact, the fitness scores turned out to be the most accurate predictor of diabetes—more than age, obesity, high blood pressure, or family history of the disease.[3]

If you don't participate in at least thirty minutes of exercise per day, talk with your doctor about ways to incorporate more exercise into your everyday life. Because of our combined experiences with helping people work out over the years, we know that most people immediately visualize exercise as just another chore, or they think it will be embarrassing, draining, or very unpleasant. So instead of exercise, try simply thinking of this as "increasing your activity level."

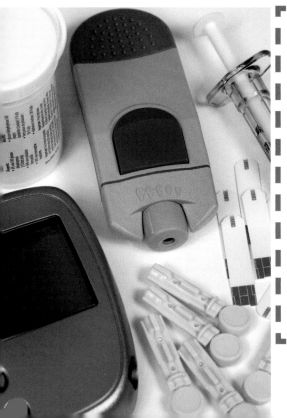

GET FIT AND LIVE!

Thigh Circumference

Thin thighs (less than 24 inches in circumference) are associated with significantly increased risk of death and cardiovascular disease. The risk increases as thigh circumference decreases. This makes it important to maintain a thigh circumference greater than 24 inches.[4]

The thigh muscles are the largest in the body and need to be exercised both aerobically and with repetitive exercises. I have found that as my patients with diabetes increase the muscle mass in their thighs, their blood sugar typically decreases.

Getting Started

Here are a few quick tips to get you started:

- First, you need to choose an activity that is fun and enjoyable. You will never stick to any activity program if you dread or hate it.

- Also, I find it is best to do your activity program with a friend or partner.

- Make sure that you wear comfortable, well-fitting shoes and socks.

- If you are a type 1 diabetic, you will need to work with your doctor in order to adjust your insulin doses while increasing your activity. Realize that exercising will lower your blood sugar; this can be potentially dangerous in a type 1 diabetic.

Aerobics and Resistance Exercises: The One-Two Punch for Type 2 Diabetes

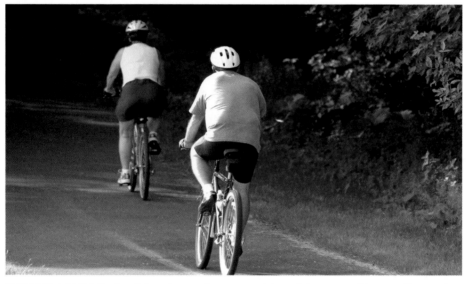

THERE IS A SIMPLE rule of thumb we often share with people who want to battle type 2 diabetes through exercise: the more muscle you build in the lower extremities and buttocks, generally the better blood sugar control you will have.

Scientific studies have proven that a combination of resistance training and aerobic exercise is the most effective way to improve insulin sensitivity in diabetics.[5] That is why we call aerobic activity and resistance training a one-two punch to knock out type 2 diabetes.

As we mentioned earlier, examples of aerobic activity are walking, cycling, swimming, working out on an elliptical machine, dancing, and hiking; it's any movement that raises the heart rate enough to help you burn fat.

We recommend simply walking in your neighborhood or a nearby park, starting with a five- or ten-minute walk, and increase it gradually as tolerated to thirty minutes or longer. Many people we work with prefer to walk for ten to fifteen minutes in the morning after breakfast and ten to fifteen minutes in the evening after dinner.

By breaking up the activity program into

two shorter time segments, most people find it easier to handle. Simply walking your dog twice a day will usually do the trick. It is also good to walk as a family after dinner and use the time to connect with each other, laugh, and unwind.

We usually start diabetics with simple resistance exercises like those we describe in chapter 7 and eventually graduate them to resistance exercises with weights. We strongly recommend starting with a certified personal trainer in order to instruct you in proper technique and to develop a good resistance program with emphasis on increasing strength and muscle mass in the lower extremities.

We find that over time most diabetics benefit from at least thirty to forty-five minutes of aerobic activity five days a week and fifteen to thirty minutes of resistance exercises three days a week. Many diabetics can perform aerobic exercises six days a week.

GET FIT AND LIVE!

Blood Sugar Control

In my type 2 diabetes patients I have found that aerobic activity combined with resistance training will improve blood sugar control even better than most diabetic medications.

Special Considerations for Diabetics

One of the best aerobic activities is simply brisk walking. However, some diabetics have foot ulcers or numbness in the feet. If this is the case with you, then walking is not the best activity for you. Instead, try cycling, the elliptical machine, or pool activities. Be sure to inspect your feet well before and after your workout session.

Perceived Exertion Scale

I used to have patients figure out their training heart rate zone and keep their heart rate in that zone. This is certainly good to do, and with new aerobic exercise equipment, one simply holds on to the handles and the machine calculates your heart rate for you. However, I've found that most diabetics hate going to a gym and simply will not exercise. For them, I recommend the perceived exertion scale. This is a scale that ranks your perceived exertion as:

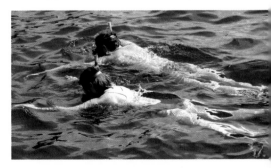

1. Very, very light
2. Very light
3. Fairly light
4. Somewhat hard
5. Very hard
6. Very, very hard

Usually, when you exercise at a perceived exertion of somewhat hard, you are typically in your target heart rate zone.

Exercises for Preventing, Slowing, and Reversing Type 2 Diabetes

YOUR LARGEST MUSCLES ARE your thighs, buttocks, and back, and we need to concentrate on these muscles. You need to focus on resistance exercises for large muscle groups that were included in the Get Fit and Live workouts in chapters 8 and 9. Specifically, make sure you include the following:

1. Squats. First do beginner squats, using a phone book on a chair, then do regular chair squats, and work up to resistance band squats or dumbbell squats.

2. Lunges with the assistance of a chair

3. Back flies with resistance bands

4. Sit-down band back flies to back row

One may eventually add the basic toning exercises if time permits.

You must also focus on aerobic exercises in the fat-burning zone.

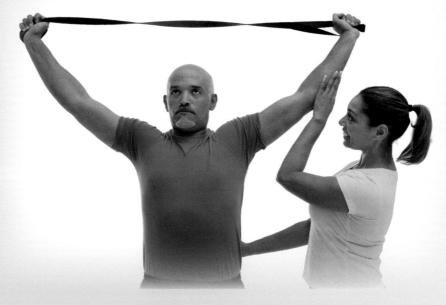

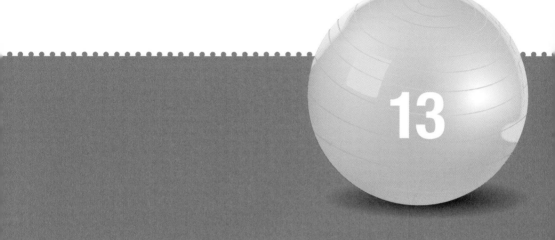

13

TARGETING OSTEOPOROSIS

TARGETING OSTEOPOROSIS

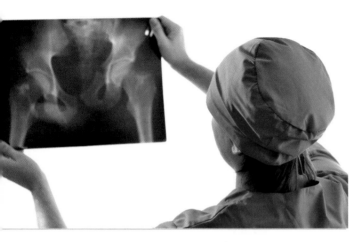

IF YOU HAVE OSTEOPO-ROSIS, you may be suffering from painful injuries caused by weak and brittle bones. But I have good news for you. God cares very deeply about you! Everything about you is important to Him, even the strength of your bones. His powerful Word says, "I will seek the lost, bring back the scattered, bind up the broken and strengthen the sick" (Ezek. 34:16, NASU). God's desire and plan for you includes renewed health and strength.

Osteoporosis can steal the strength from your bones, leaving you stoop-shouldered and prone to fractures. But there is something you can do to help lower your risk for a break—you can exercise!

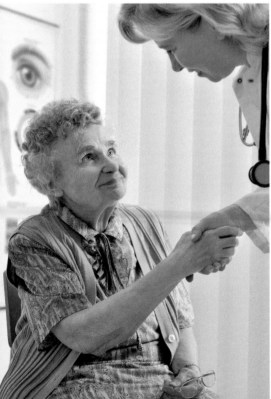

Benefits of Exercise in Fighting Osteoporosis

Exercise can help prevent osteoporosis, and it can help treat it by providing strength to your bones and muscles. Exercise will slow mineral loss, help you maintain posture, and improve your overall fitness, which reduces the risk of falls.

Building Muscle Is the Key

Weight-bearing exercises and strengthening exercises are the most important forms of exercise in treating osteoporosis. However, using weights or calisthenics to build muscles will also help to build bones. Realize the stronger your muscles are, generally the stronger your bones are. For more information on this topic, please refer to the book *The New Bible Cure for Osteoporosis*.

Get Moving!

The sedentary lifestyle common in America is one of the greatest risks for eventually developing osteoporosis. Why? Because the human bone is constantly being remodeled and reformed, and this remodeling happens in response to the demands and stresses that are placed on the bone *by exercise*.

Weight-bearing exercises will actually stimulate the growth of new bone cells. The bones, however, must be stressed in order to grow. Weight-bearing exercise will not only stop bone loss but will also increase the mass of bone.

A sedentary lifestyle is death to your bones. We have seen many women develop osteoporosis, and many of these women have had adequate amounts of calcium in their diets. But they don't stress their bones adequately through exercise, and, as a result, they lose significant amounts of bone. (Men also lose bone mass as they age, but typically not to the same degree as women.)

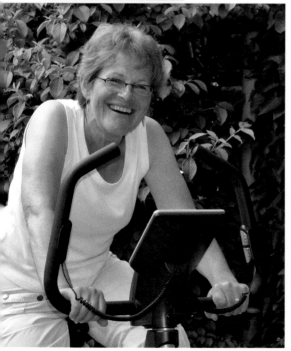

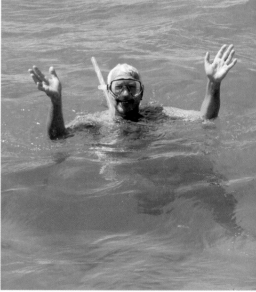

WEIGHT-BEARING EXERCISES

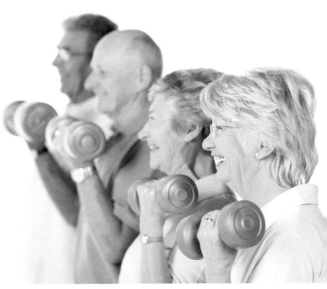

WHICH EXERCISES WILL PREVENT osteoporosis? Many doctors encourage swimming and cycling, and these are wonderful exercises for improving your overall health. However, these exercises will not prevent osteoporosis. Only weight-bearing exercises will stimulate bone growth.[1] Cycling will stress the leg bones, but it will do nothing to stress the entire skeleton. Swimming puts no stress on the skeleton whatsoever and will not prevent osteoporosis.

Weight-bearing exercises such as dancing, walking, running, stair climbing, team sports, and yard work are often recommended in fighting osteoporosis. They are beneficial because they will stress (and thereby strengthen) the leg bones and hip bones. However, these activities are not as beneficial in preventing osteoporosis in the upper body—the spine, arms, and so forth.

The only exercises that prevent osteoporosis in the entire skeleton are weight-bearing exercises such as weight lifting and calisthenics. It's a well-known fact that, on average, weight lifters' bones are much thicker than those who don't lift weights. We highly encourage you to begin a weight-lifting routine that will stress all of the major bones in your body and thus stimulate growth.

Perhaps you really don't think weight lifting is your thing, or you need a "no-cost" program. Don't worry! Performing calisthenics such as push-ups, lunges, squats, seated dips, or even lifting a five-pound bag of sugar, a can of paint, or a gallon of bottled water over your head long way in improving your bone health.

Think About Hiring a Certified Personal Trainer

On the next page, we are about to describe several simple weight-lifting exercises that will benefit your bones. However, you may find it very helpful to join a gym and have a certified personal trainer demonstrate weight-lifting exercises that will prevent osteoporosis.

A gym and trainer might be beyond your budget right now. If so, a "low-cost" option is to buy dumbbells and and the equipment recommended on page 68 at Sports Authority or Play It Again Sports and begin a basic weight-lifting program right in your own home.

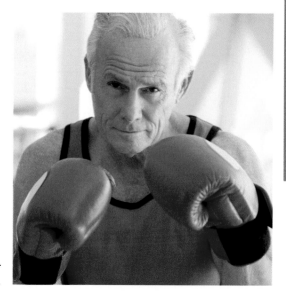

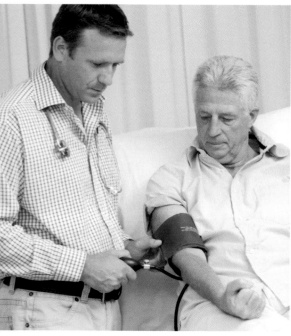

Don't Forget to Check With Your Doctor

It's very important to know which exercises will benefit you and which ones you as an individual need to avoid. Never begin an exercise program—especially if you already have osteoporosis—without checking with your doctor first. Your doctor will determine if you are ready for a bone-strengthening program. Some patients have such severe osteoporosis that they are at a high fracture risk and shouldn't exercise until their condition is stabilized.

If you've checked with your doctor, then you can begin doing some of these exercises right away. So, turn the page!

EXERCISES TO FIGHT OSTEOPOROSIS

OSTEOPOROSIS PRIMARILY AFFECTS THE bones of the spine, hips, and forearms. Therefore, exercises tailored to prevent further loss to these three groups of bones are extremely important. Do these exercises approximately three times a week.

Overhead presses

While seated or standing, simply take a pair of five- or ten-pound dumbbells and lift them over your head five to ten times. Repeat this for two to three sets.

Lunges

To perform lunges, start by performing the lunges with a chair (as shown) for a few months. Then add hand weights for a few months and eventually incorporate dumbbells. To incorporate weights or dumbbells, simply hold the weights or dumbbells down by your side and step forward with one foot and lunge outward. Then come back to a standing position with your feet together. Start with a comfortable number of repetitions like two or three, and eventually increase the number as you are comfortable. Your goal should be eight to twelve reps.

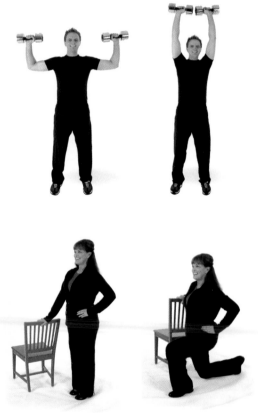

Squats

To perform squats, start with a chair (as shown) for a few weeks or months and eventually incorporate dumbbells or resistance bands. To add dumbbells or resistance bands, hold the dumbbells or bands at your sides. If using bands, the bands should be under your feet. With legs apart, simply squat down. Start with a comfortable number of repetitions, like two or three. Increase the number as you are comfortable and eventually work up to eight to twelve reps. If chair squats are too difficult, simply put a thick phone book on the chair. As your thighs get stronger, remove the phone book.

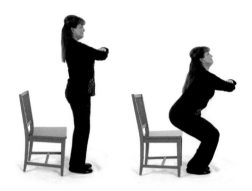

Push-ups

Push-ups are great for the forearms and arms. However, many women cannot perform them. I recommend doing push-ups from the knees instead of from the feet. Performing these simple exercises will help you to prevent further bone loss. Start with a comfortable number of repetitions like two or three. Increase the number as you are comfortable, and eventually work up to eight to twelve reps.

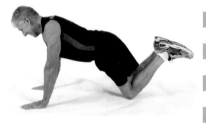

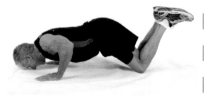

14

TARGETING FIBROMYALGIA AND CHRONIC FATIGUE

Fibromyalgia and Chronic Fatigue Syndrome

PEOPLE WITH FIBROMYALGIA AND chronic fatigue syndrome usually hate to exercise since first of all they are usually exhausted and patients with fibromyalgia have painful trigger points throughout their body causing very tender muscles. However, we can promise you that nothing is more invigorating than practicing a regular exercise routine.

The apostle Paul said, "I discipline my body like an athlete, training it to do what it should. Otherwise, I fear that after preaching to others I myself might be disqualified" (1 Cor. 9:27). Like the apostle Paul, we believe in the powerful benefits of exercise. Regular, daily exercise can help to eliminate the effects of stress, which is another major cause of chronic fatigue and fibromyalgia.

Resting or relaxing during the day and taking a nap is also very beneficial for relieving stress. When you are resting or relaxing, you may want to listen to a relaxation tape or calm, soothing music and practice deep-breathing exercises. Rest and relaxation are just as important as the rest of your exercise routine because they help to counter the effects of stress.

The exercises we recommend in this chapter will help you to overcome the fatigue caused by excessive stress over a long period of time. On this page are some basic steps you can take to help overcome even the most severe fatigue. If your fatigue is less severe, please be sure to read the section "Ready for More?" on page 154.

Dr. Colbert Approved

Breathing Exercises

I highly recommend that you practice abdominal breathing. Chest breathing tends to be more shallow and rapid and is commonly practiced when a person is under stress. However, abdominal breathing, which involves moving the abdominal muscles outward, has been shown to be the best form of breathing to relieve stress.

In order to learn abdominal breathing, it is best to lie on your back and place a large book on the abdomen, such as a dictionary or large family Bible. While brea move the abdomen outward, thus causing book to rise higher in the air. Concentrate on moving the abdon outward and not expanding the rib cage.

As this is practiced, you will be able to perform abdomir breathing while sitting, standing, or walking. When you fe stressed, perform five or ten slow, deep, abdominal breaths relax your body.

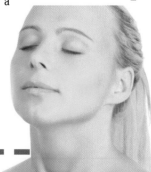

Progressive Muscle Relaxation Exercises

Practice this when you are reclining in a comfortable chair, on a bed, or on the couch. Close your eyes to relax. Beginning with the feet, tense the toes by curling them under; hold this position for five seconds and then relax. As you relax, simply let the tension leave your body.

Next, flex the ankle joint. Pull the toes back while flexing the calf muscle. Again, hold this position for five seconds and then relax. Next, point the toes like a ballerina, and again flex the calf for five seconds and relax. Move to the legs and flex the thighs tight. Hold this for five seconds and relax.

Gradually working your way up your body, flex the muscles in the abdomen, arms, chest, shoulders, hands, neck, forehead, eyes, and jaw. Once again, do each of these for five seconds and then relax. The tension will melt away.

Special Considerations for Those With Chronic Fatigue

If you suffer from chronic fatigue syndrome, you may feel too exhausted to even think about jogging at this point, but what about walking? Slow walking is the best exercise to start with. If you are unable to walk, simply perform the stretching exercises in chapter 10.

Do something you love and start slowly, gradually building your exercise routine. If you love the outdoors, take a slow walk through your favorite park. Also walk in a mall slowly and window shop. Start with a five-minute walk and gradually increase your speed and time as tolerated. Some people will need to exercise every other day instead of daily. Do not try to push yourself too fast, or it may make your fatigue or fibromyalgia worse. Many prefer to walk for five minutes twice a day rather than ten minutes once a day. Eventually, work your way up to a ten-minute walk, twice a day if you are able, but do not push yourself too fast.

A Word of Caution

If you have been under continual, chronic stress for many years and feel totally exhausted, you may have very low adrenal function. If simple brisk walking causes exhaustion, then you should refrain from doing this form of exercise until your adrenal function has been restored. Rest and take the supplements recommended in the books *The Bible Cure for Chronic Fatigue and Fibromyalgia* and *Stress Less*. Most patients will benefit from adrenal rebuilder supplements, pregnenolone, and adaptogens. Once your adrenal function is completely restored, you will be able to perform moderate exercise without exhaustion.

Never push yourself if you feel exhausted after exercise. You could further weaken your adrenal glands and cause even more severe fatigue. Use balance and wisdom.

READY FOR MORE?

YOUR FATIGUE MAY NOT be at a severe level. If so, you may be able to skip the building stages discussed on the previous pages and get into more vigorous exercise. We typically recommend that you exercise for ten to twenty minutes every other day at 65 percent of your maximum heart rate (see page 33 to determine your heart rate) when battling mild fibromyalgia and mild chronic fatigue.

The key exercise for chronic fatigue and fibromyalgia is stretching and aerobic movement, and NOT strengthening exercises. The strengthening exercises come much later when the fatigue and painful trigger points of fibromyalgia are resolved. Toning and strengthening exercises will many times worsen both chronic fatigue and fibromyalgia. The reason is that fibromyalgia patients already have painful trigger points or muscle spasms, and toning and strengthening exercises will typically make these worse.

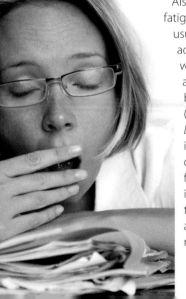

Also, chronic fatigue patients usually have adrenal fatigue, which is like an overdrawn bank account (refer to *Stress Less* for more information on adrenal fatigue). Toning and resistance exercises and even too much aerobic exercise will further deplete their energy levels or adrenal reserve, possibly making their symptoms worse.

Therefore, the correct type of exercise and the proper frequency of exercise needs are dependent on the severity of the chronic fatigue syndrome or fibromyalgia. Most patients with chronic fatigue syndrome and fibromyalgia will benefit from daily stretching exercises. Please refer to the basic stretching exercises in chapter 10. We typically recommend that you perform aerobic exercises every other day, depending on your symptoms. Some people can only perform aerobic exercises once or twice a week because these exercises deplete their energy. Many can only perform five or ten minutes of aerobic exercise and not the twenty to thirty minutes that we typically recommend. And that is OK because as you perform the stretching exercises, you will improve lymphatic flow and help to relax your muscles, which should improve your condition.

Gently jumping on a minitrampoline (a rebounder) for one to five minutes, one or two times a day is very good for people with chronic fatigue syndrome and fibromyalgia, since it improves lymphatic flow. (See pages 164–165 for instructions on rebounding.)

1. See basic stretches in chapter 10.
2. Add the other stretches from the FREE downloadable video that accompanies this book.

You Could Have an Undiagnosed Infection

Many chronic fatigue patients and fibromyalgia patients have undiagnosed chronic viral infections such as EBV (Epstein-Barr virus), CMV (cytomegalo virus), and HHV-6 (human herpesvirus 6). Also, quite a few may have Lyme disease. So be sure to have your doctor check for these diseases.

The Trigger Points of Fibromyalgia

The repressed emotions I discuss in the sidebar on this page can create muscle tension that constricts the blood vessels supplying oxygen to the muscles in the trigger point areas, reducing the blood supply and oxygen to the muscles. The result is painful trigger points that can lead to numbness, the sensation of pins and needles, and even decreased strength in the muscles. Patients with both chronic fatigue and fibromyalgia also usually have lymphatic stasis from lack of movement and painful trigger points.

GET FIT and LIVE!

If You Have Trouble Sleeping...

Aerobic exercise, such as walking, swimming, or cycling, will usually improve the quality of sleep. Regular aerobic exercise helps the body to make smooth transitions between sleep cycles and stages of sleep.

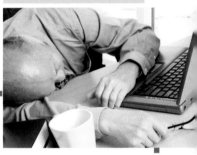

Dr. Colbert Approved

Discovering the Emotional Connection to Your Pain

I have found that many of my fibromyalgia patients have repressed anger and unforgiveness. As a result, I have had amazing success in treating fibromyalgia by taking patients through what I call "forgiveness therapy." (For more information on forgiveness therapy, refer to my books *Stress Less* and *The Seven Pillars of Health*.)

If you feel that repressed emotions may be expressing themselves through your fibromyalgia, be encouraged. Even if your pain has been around for years, there's so much you can begin to do to get genuine relief from your pain. I believe that you did not pick up this book by accident. God sees your pain and understands it far better than you ever could. Not only does He understand you, but He is also your heavenly Father who loves you.

He wants to help you uncover the roots of your pain, and He will bring lasting healing and relief. As you come to Jesus Christ, your weary soul will find blessed rest from the raging storms of physical pain and fatigue. Why not bow your head right now and turn over your spiritual pain to Jesus? If you've never invited Jesus Christ to be a part of your life, I encourage you to turn to the back of this book, where I've written a special message that will introduce you to Him.

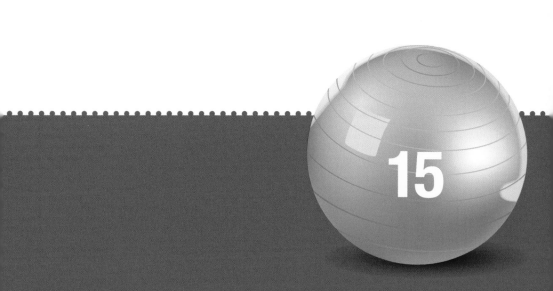

15

TARGETING HEART DISEASE

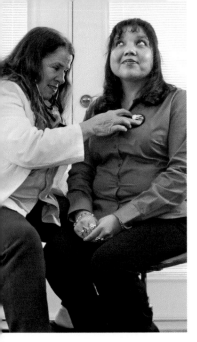

TARGETING A HEALTHY HEART

BY FAR THE MOST important exercise for the heart is aerobic exercise in the fat-burning zone or target heart rate zone. Also, the longer and the more consistent you are at performing the aerobic exercise, usually the better off you are. We usually instruct people to start training aerobically for five or ten minutes a day at around 65 percent of their predicted maximum heart rate. We then gradually increase their time every week or so to fifteen minutes, then twenty minutes, then twenty-five minutes, and so on up to forty-five to sixty minutes, five days a week. Realize that consistent aerobic exercise for longer periods of time increases your HDL cholesterol (good cholesterol).

What's Your Fat-Burning Zone?

Your fat-burning zone is the lower end of your target heart rate zone, meaning you should stay within 65–70 percent of your maximum heart rate. (See page 33 to learn how to calculate your heart rate.)

Weight Lifters Beware!

Unfortunately, many weight lifters and bodybuilders are lifting heavy weights and straining and holding their breath with each repetition. This tends to raise the blood pressure and contribute to heart disease.

Sadly, we've personally witnessed middle-aged men suffer both heart attacks and strokes while lifting weights in the gym. That is the reason why we do not recommend lifting heavy weights and why we recommend you breathe properly and never hold your breath and strain while lifting since this usually raises your blood pressure.

Now we do recommend calisthenics, resistance band exercises, or lifting lighter weights with more repetitions, along with proper breathing, in order to tone the muscles and not raise the blood pressure. Most weight lifters and bodybuilders are neglecting the most important muscle in their body, and this is the heart.

Slow and Steady Wins the Race

Exercise gets the heart pumping, right? So if you exercise regularly, will you overwork your heart? The answer is no. Ironically, *inactivity* puts more mileage on your heart than an active lifestyle. Why? Because an inactive person's heart is unconditioned and less efficient, and therefore, it must work much harder (80 or more beats per minute) than an active person's heart (60 to 70 beats per minute). And a slower heart is a healthier heart. Having a slower pulse means your heart has more time to feed itself with oxygen between beats. The longer the pause from beat to beat, the more nourishment your heart gets from your blood.

See Your Doctor First

If you have multiple cardiovascular risk factors such as hypertension (high blood pressure), smoking, high cholesterol, or a family history of heart disease, I strongly recommend that you get a physical examination and undergo an exercise stress test before beginning an exercise program.

Every year in the United States about 75,000 heart attacks are brought on by heavy exertion such as vigorous exercise. People with a sedentary lifestyle who have risk factors for heart attack are at the greatest risk. Therefore, even after your physician has cleared you for exercise, I recommend you avoid intense exercise until your cardiovascular risk factors have been modified and your heart fitness has improved. Studies show that after one year of regular activity, your risks of heart attack are greatly reduced and exercise becomes protective for your heart.[1]

GET FIT AND LIVE!

Cut Your Risk in Half!

In a study where researchers monitored over 84,000 nurses for eight years, the nurses who exercised regularly had a 54 percent lower risk of both heart attack and stroke when compared to sedentary women.[2] That's a good reason to get moving! (And exercise costs less than Lipitor, the leading cholesterol-lowering medication, which costs more than three dollars per tablet.)

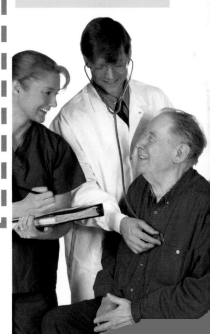

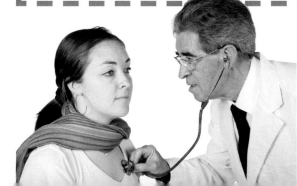

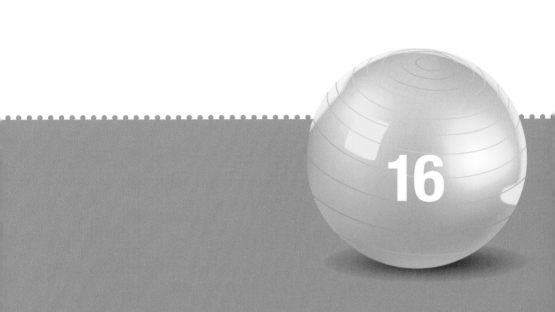

TARGETING CANCER

TARGETING CANCER

THE BEST FORM OF exercise for fighting cancer is aerobic exercise, which includes brisk walking, cycling, swimming, or jogging. Some doctors say that just thirty minutes of exercise every other day can reduce the risk of breast cancer by 75 percent. You see, cancer cells are anaerobic, which means they don't thrive in high-oxygen environments. Exercise pumps oxygen to your cells, giving your body added ability to win the war against cancer.

Beginning a fitness routine can be challenging for a healthy person; it may be even harder for you if you are in the midst of cancer treatment. The key is to start slow and increase frequency or intensity gradually as you are able. Keep activity periods short, and take frequent breaks for rest and replenishment of liquids. For example, divide a twenty-minute walk into two ten-minute intervals, allowing time to take a breather and drink some water during breaks. If you are too tired to walk for ten minutes, you may want to stick to ten minutes of stretching instead. Turn to the next page for our specific exercise recommendations.

Workouts for Keeping Cancer Away

How often do you exercise during the week? Did you know that getting out and jogging, walking, or bicycling—or participating in any type of regular, moderate form of exertion—can help you avoid cancer or keep it from coming back? It's time to get up off the couch and get active! According to the American Medical Association, people who exercise regularly have lower incidences of cancer in general. My favorite exercises to recommend for cancer patients are aerobic exercise such as walking and rebounding (jumping on a minitrampoline). Turn the page for complete rebounding workout instructions.

Dr. Colbert Approved

Exercise Can Benefit Cancer Patients[1]

According to the American Cancer Society (ACS), regular moderate exercise has been found to have health benefits for those fighting cancer. The following are all possible benefits of regular exercise during cancer treatment listed on the ACS Web site. Exercise can:

- Improve your physical abilities
- Lower your risk of falls and broken bones by helping you maintain balance
- Keep your muscles from wasting due to inactivity
- Maintain better blood flow to legs and lower the risk of blood clots
- Improve your self-esteem
- Lower your risk of anxiety and depression
- Lessen nausea

Cautions for Cancer Patients[2]

There are many variables that can affect your ability to work out while you are overcoming cancer, so it is critical that you only take on activities your doctor or cancer team has approved. Be sure to talk to them first if you have questions about any of the following. The ACS warns against exercising if:

- You have a low red blood cell count (anemia) or low white blood cell count
- You have a low amount of sodium and potassium in your blood, which can happen if you are frequently vomiting or have diarrhea
- You have numbness in your feet, which can cause you to fall
- You are on blood thinners (you should avoid any activity that increases your risk of falling)
- You still have a catheter (tube) inserted in your body
- You are experiencing nausea or vomiting

You should contact your doctor right away if you experience any of the following while exercising:

- Swollen ankles
- Shortness of breath, especially if this occurs while at rest or with minimal exertion
- Pain
- Dizziness
- Blurred vision

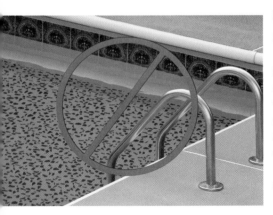

Special Cancer Conditions[3]

Bones: Don't exercise with heavy weights if you have cancer that has spread to the bone or you have other health conditions that could weaken your bones, such as osteoporosis. Any exercise that puts too much stress on the bones could put you at serious risk of breaking a bone or other injury.

Skin: Don't swim in chlorinated pools if your skin has had radiation treatment. The chlorine may cause irritation.

SEVEN-MINUTE REBOUNDING ROUTINE

THERE ARE MANY BENEFITS of rebounding (bouncing on a minitrampoline). It increases circulation; improves coordination, balance, and agility; burns about three hundred calories per hour; and is easier on your joints than jogging or walking. But the main benefit of rebounding is its helpfulness in combating cancer due to its effect on the body's lymphatic system. Vigorous exercise such as rebounding is reported to increase lymph flow by fifteen to thirty times.[4] Here's our seven-minute rebounding routine that will help you fight cancer and improve your overall health.

Starting stance

Step onto the rebounder, and center yourself with feet shoulder width apart and hands at your sides. Keep your knees slightly bent and stomach tight.

TIP: Look straight ahead at something that doesn't move on your horizon, rather than looking down at your feet.

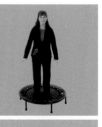

Two-Minute Warm-Up Walk

Place your hands on your hips and alternate stepping with each foot to mimic walking in place, keeping your feet shoulder width apart. Keep your stomach tight and your breathing even as you warm up.

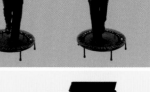

One-Minute Light Bounce

Start a gentle bounce with both feet, keeping your knees slightly bent and keeping both feet in contact with the rebounder at all times. Bounce by pressing down into the rebounder rather than jumping up off of it.

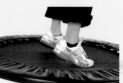

One-Minute Get-Fit Bounce

Keep the bouncing in a gentle rhythm, but begin to heighten your bounce and lift off of the rebounder. Keep your focus on regular breathing and tightening your core (abdomen).

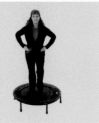

One-Minute Get-Fit Bounce With Arm Raise

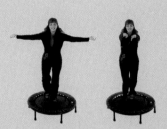

Keep bouncing as described in the Get-Fit Bounce, but raise your arms to shoulder height, holding them straight out to your sides. Bounce ten to twelve times. Now bring your arms straight out in front of you, keeping them at shoulder height, palms facing down. Bounce ten to twelve times. Keep alternating arm positions for ten to twelve bounces until the minute is up. You can also alternate facing your palms up and facing your palms down.

TIP: If balance is a challenge, you can raise one arm at a time while holding onto a stabilizer bar with the other hand.

One-Minute Get-Fit Bounce With High Knees

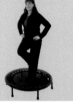

Keeping your feet shoulder width apart, place your hands on your hips as you bounce. Alternate lifting your knees to your chest (or as high as you can) while you bounce. Push down into the rebounder with the heel of your foot while you raise the alternate knee.

One-Minute Cool-Down Walk

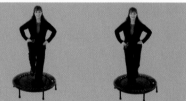

Repeat the warm-up walk as a cooldown. Breathe deeply, and keep your core (stomach) tight as you slow your pace down to a walk.

Important Rebounding Tips

- To avoid the risk of prolapsed organs, beginners should stick to the "Light Bounce" described on the previous page, keeping your feet in contact with the rebounder at all times. Do this for about three to five minutes per session. (Seniors should start with two minutes per session.) You can have more than one session per day as long as you wait at least thirty minutes in between sessions. You can increase the length of time as your fitness improves.

- Some rebounders come with an optional stability bar. I recommend using one if keeping your balance on the rebounder is a challenge. You can also place the rebounder near a wall and lean on the wall as you step on and off of the rebounder.

- Either wear athletic shoes or go barefoot on your rebounder. Don't jump in stocking feet because you will be more likely to slip.

- For an advanced option, add weights as you become stronger and more skilled at rebounding.

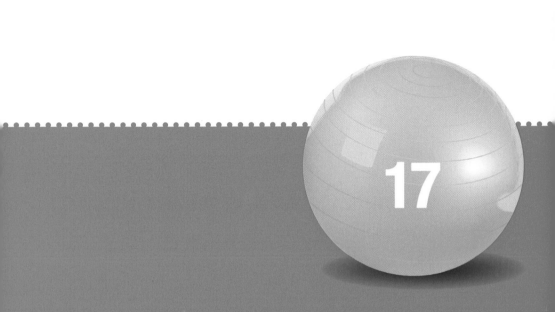

TARGETING ARTHRITIS

Exercises That Help You Beat Osteoarthritis

WHILE PHYSICAL EXERCISE MAY be painful at first, it is an essential ingredient in God's plan for you to overcome arthritis. Exercise not only decreases the risk of developing heart disease, cancer, hypertension, diabetes, and osteoporosis, but it also decreases the risk of developing osteoarthritis and helps to slow the progression of osteoarthritis. In other words, exercise helps prevent most degenerative diseases. The sidebar on this page lists the various ways exercise can benefit you if you suffer from osteoarthritis.

Ways That Exercise Prevents Osteoarthritis

1. Exercise lubricates your cartilage.

Just as oil lubricates the moving parts of an engine, synovial fluid serves the function of lubricating cartilage. An adequate supply of synovial fluid will actually help prevent or slow down the development of osteoarthritis. Exercise helps to improve the flow of synovial fluid into and out of the cartilage. This in turn keeps the cartilage healthy and moist and prevents the drying and thinning of the cartilage that is so often seen in osteoarthritis. It is extremely important for the synovial fluid to keep the cartilage moist in order to prevent frictional forces that dry out the cartilage and cause wear and tear and thinning.

2. Exercising helps you reach and maintain your ideal weight.

This is one of the best preventive measures for osteoarthritis. Obesity and excess body weight are associated with increased stress on the weight-bearing joints, which will eventually trigger osteoarthritis.

3. Exercise helps maintain the range of motion of your joints.

The less a joint is used, the less range of motion you will maintain. An example of this is when a patient develops a painful shoulder and, due to the pain, will not use the shoulder. He will not reach overhead or exercise the shoulder through a full range of motion. Within one to three weeks, he may develop a frozen shoulder and be unable to extend his arm overhead or adequately rotate his shoulder. By not using the shoulder on a daily basis, he will actually lose the function of the shoulder. In other words, exercise maintains the flexibility of the joint. Avoidance of exercise can severely limit the normal range of motion of a joint.

4. Exercise strengthens your tendons, ligaments, and muscles.

The tendons, ligaments, and muscles that support your joints are strengthened through regular exercise. This in turn adds more protection for your joints by absorbing the majority of the force placed on the joints.

Each time you exercise, you put pressure on the joints. The majority of the pressure is absorbed by the supporting structures, including the muscles, ligaments, and tendons.

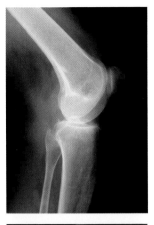

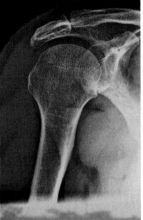

Since cartilage has no blood vessels, the cartilage relies on an exchange of fluid through the synovial fluid in order to take in nutrients and eliminate waste products. Exercise encourages this process of taking in nutrients into the cartilage through the synovial fluid and expelling waste products or toxic material out of the cartilage.

Getting Ready to Begin

Here are a few things to keep in mind as you get fit to overcome arthritis:

Consult a physician.

Some exercises, like jogging and running, can actually worsen arthritis, while others, such as cycling, pool exercises, and exercise on an elliptical machine, can greatly improve it. Be sure to consult with your doctor or physical therapist before starting any exercise program. You should also be screened to rule out significant cardiovascular disease before beginning the aerobic exercise I recommend on the next page.

Use a heart rate monitor.

Prior to beginning an aerobic exercise program, you may want to purchase a heart rate monitor, and you should calculate your training heart rate.

Train within your heart rate zone.

Refer to page 33 for the formula to help you train within your target heart rate. We recommend training within the lower range, 65–70 percent, or the fat-burning zone.

Drink adequate water.

Adequate hydration and exercise are probably the two most important components in assuring adequate flow of the synovial fluid into and out of the cartilage.

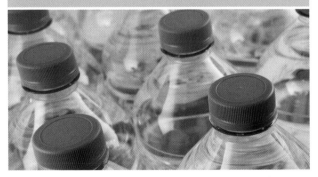

EXERCISES FOR OSTEOARTHRITIS

Weight-bearing exercises

Weight-bearing exercises are some of the best forms of exercise for mild arthritis sufferers. However, if your arthritis is moderate to severe, you should start with non-weight-bearing exercises such as pool exercises or water aerobics and gradually work into weight-bearing exercises. Weight-bearing exercises are simply exercises where you are actually working against the force of gravity, such as walking, using stair steppers and elliptical machines, and low-impact aerobics. Weight-bearing exercises help the bones grow stronger and thicker. However, this form of exercise is most effective for the lower part of the body, especially the ankles, knees, hips, and lower back, more so than the upper body.

Weight lifting

Lifting light weights and performing other calisthenic or isotonic types of exercises are also important in helping to build strong bones and muscles and to help prevent or slow the progress of osteoarthritis. You should lift light weights at very slow speeds, maintaining good form, and perform at least eight to twelve repetitions a set. To avoid injury, seek a certified personal trainer to instruct you on the proper techniques in lifting weights.

Walking

If you are interested in preventing arthritis, simply getting out and walking is a great way to keep the tendons, ligaments, and muscles that support your joints in proper working order. However, if you already suffer from moderate to severe arthritis, you may be unable to walk sufficient distances to adequately work your muscles. Therefore, I recommend alternative low-impact aerobic exercises such as cycling and using an elliptical machine for those who are already dealing with this degenerative disease.

Alternative low-impact aerobic exercises

These exercises include ballroom dancing, tai chi, and hatha yoga. They take the strain off of the joints while at the same time strengthening the supporting structures, tendons, and ligaments and stimulating the flow of the synovial fluid in the joints. I recommend that my arthritic patients perform aerobic exercise three to four times a week for at least twenty minutes. (Often, my patients need to start at five minutes and gradually work up to twenty minutes by increasing the length of time every week or two.)

Stretching

Stretching exercises are also very important for both preventing arthritis and improving flexibility in arthritic joints. Stretching increases your flexibility, improves the range of motion of a joint, and makes you less prone to injury during weight-lifting exercises.

Exercise Routine for Arthritis

- In starting an exercise program, it is best to warm up for five to ten minutes on a stationary bike, elliptical machine, or treadmill.

- After you have adequately warmed your muscles up, then stretch anywhere from five to ten minutes.

- After stretching, lift light weights or perform calisthenic exercises for approximately twenty to thirty minutes. (We recommend weight machines rather than free weights since you are less likely to injure yourself with the machines.)

- After working out with weights, perform an aerobic exercise for twenty minutes at the lower end of your training heart rate.

- Finish up by stretching slowly and holding the movement at the end of the stretch for approximately one to two seconds.* Count one-one thousand, two-one thousand, and then release the stretch. Perform anywhere from ten to twenty repetitions per movement. Some basic stretches include neck, back, knee, hip, and leg stretches.

---

* If you develop pain in your joints, stop stretching in this manner.

GET FIT AND LIVE!

Get Fit and Get Rid . . . of Meds

Many of my arthritic patients who begin to exercise on a regular basis improve so much that I am able to decrease their medications or even eliminate them entirely!

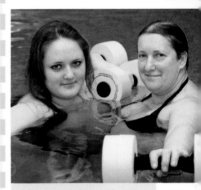

Aquatic Exercise Helps *Both* Types of Arthritis

Some forms of exercise benefit one form of arthritis but not the other. But aquatic exercise (water aerobics) benefits *both* types of arthritis—osteoarthritis and rheumatoid arthritis—because it is much easier on joints and muscles.

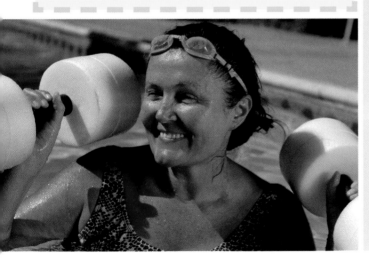

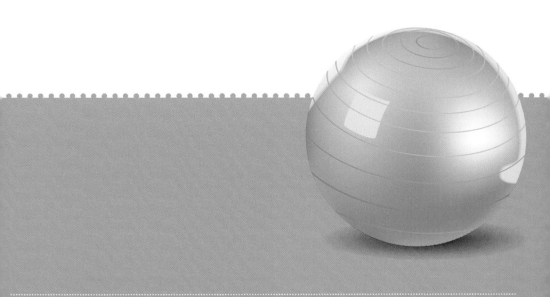

CONCLUSION

HOW TO SUCCEED AT GETTING FIT

HEALTH CLUBS KNOW A secret: most exercisers drop out. Clubs sign up more people than can use their facilities, knowing that many people who pay for membership won't show up. The health club pencil pushers are right. Our experiences as a doctor and personal trainer have taught us that people often start well, then quit exercising. Think about all the unused exercise equipment lying under beds, under sheets in the guest bedroom, and in garages across America. Big chains like Play It Again Sports thrive on good intentions that never take hold.

Your body will not do the right thing without some prodding. It doesn't like being exercised at first, but after about three weeks your body will change its mind: it will desire and expect to exercise. The sidebar on the next page contains the best tips we know to bulletproof your exercise routine.

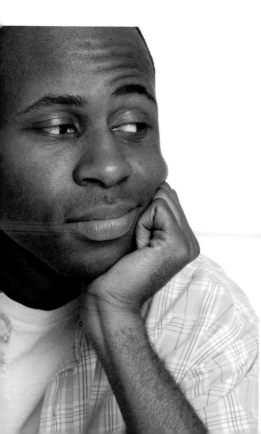

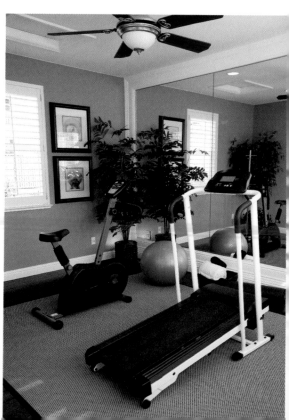

How to Bulletproof Your Exercise Routine

GET FIT AND LIVE!

- Build exercise into your schedule. Schedule it like an important doctor's appointment. Choose a time you won't waver from, and put yourself on automatic so you don't give yourself an "out."

- A workout before breakfast, before lunch, or before dinner is great. Just don't exercise late at night since you may be too charged up to sleep. Also, avoid exercise immediately after a meal. It will pull the blood from your stomach and intestines (where it's needed to help digestion) to your muscles. You are likely to start belching and to have heartburn and other digestive problems. Exercise before you eat or two hours after you eat. However, a light snack before exercising is fine.

- Choose an exercise you enjoy. The best exercise is the one you'll do. If you have arthritis and walking hurts your knees, choose biking, elliptical machines, pool exercises, yoga, or tai chi instead. Tailor your routine to your physical condition.

- Have an exercise partner. Partners keep you accountable to do the exercise and should make the exercise time more enjoyable.

- Choose a location you enjoy. Walk in malls, parks, mountains, on the beach, or near a lake. Make exercise a complete sensory experience.

- Change it up. Change your routine either by location, time of day, or by the exercise you do. Make it fun.

- Do occupational/transportation exercises. Seize every opportunity to increase your activity level. Park at the far end of the parking lot and walk to the store. Use stairs when you can. Default to the active option.

Quick Quiz
Walk the Dog—and Lose Weight

In a university study, people who walked their dog for twenty minutes a day, five days a week, lost how many pounds after one year?

- 4 pounds
- 9 pounds
- 14 pounds
- 22 pounds

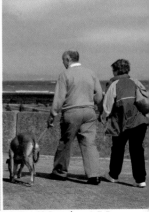

Answer: c. 14 pounds. According to a University of Missouri–Columbia study, participants, none of whom were regular walkers before the study, began by walking dogs ten minutes per day, three times each week, and worked up to twenty minutes per day, five times each week. Those who followed this program for fifty weeks lost an average of fourteen pounds. Those who walked only twenty-six weeks didn't see significant weight loss.[1]

TAKING CUES FROM YOUR BODY

IT'S IMPORTANT TO TAKE a rest when needed. On days when you are exhausted, or after nights in which you have not slept well, don't push yourself to exercise. Listen to your body, and learn when to take a day off.

We have talked at length with many highly trained athletes, including marathon runners, who are compulsive exercise enthusiasts. The downside of compulsive exercise is that many of these people suffer from constant muscle soreness from overtraining and chronic fatigue. By contrast, we recommend low-intensity workouts and moderation in physical exertion, because the pressure associated with excessive exercise can undo the very thing you are trying to accomplish.

It's important to get your heartbeat up to your target heart rate zone or fat-burning zone (see page 33), but exercising as hard as you can is like flooring the accelerator of your car. It's not good for the engine. When you push your body too hard, you release tremendous amounts of free radicals into your system that can damage cells, tissues, and even organs. The increase of free radicals also accelerates the aging process.

Overtraining can suppress your immune system, increase your risk of injury, increase your body fat by raising cortisol levels, and interfere with your emotional and mental health. It can cause as much stress to the body as trauma, surgery, infections, and anxiety.

Are You Overtraining?

Examples of overtraining include:

- Spending hours on a treadmill, running off the stress of a hard day
- Pushing yourself to lift heavier weights for more repetitions even though your strength is diminishing
- Training at a heart rate over 90 percent of your target heart rate or starting out exercising at over 80 percent of your target heart rate
- Lifting weights for too long, at too high intensity, at one session or for too many days in a row. It's generally best to lift weights every other day to let your muscles recuperate.

With these tips you should have everything you need to find an enjoyable way to stir the waters of life with exercise.

Avoiding Muscle Pain After Exercise

Delayed onset muscle soreness (DOMS) after exercise is common when you begin an exercise program. You might feel stiff and sore in the hours and days after you exercise. Here are tips to treat and avoid muscle soreness:[2]

- Warm up thoroughly five minutes before activity, and cool down completely three to five minutes afterward.

- Perform easy stretching after exercise.

- When beginning a new activity, start gradually and build up your time and intensity over time.

- Avoid making sudden major changes in the type of exercises you do.

- Avoid making sudden major changes in the amount of time that you exercise.

- Wait. Soreness will go away in three to seven days with no special treatment.

- Do some easy, low-impact aerobic exercise—this will increase blood flow to the affected muscles, which may help diminish soreness.

- Gently stretch the affected area.

- Gently massage the affected muscles.

Whatever aerobic exercise you do, gradually increase the time and intensity, going from five minutes to ten, then eventually up to thirty or even forty minutes. Drink plenty of water to replace what you are losing through sweat and exhalation. Avoid exercising immediately after a meal, because exercise triggers the body to carry blood away from your stomach and intestines to your muscles, which impairs digestion. Wait at least two hours after you eat before exercising unless you eat only a light snack.

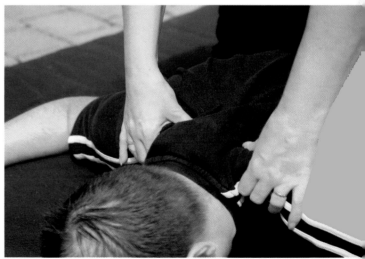

STICKING WITH IT

MANY PEOPLE FIND THAT, difficult as it is to start an exercise program, it is even more difficult to stick with it. Here's a tip: make your walking program a vital part of your day. Too many people get into trouble when they save exercising for their spare time. If you wait until you can get around to it, you probably never will.

Choose an exercise activity that you truly enjoy. Walking is only one suggestion. Have you tried ballroom dancing? Or backpacking? Perhaps you've always pictured yourself on a tennis court. Surely there is an activity that you always thought you'd like to try. Now's the time—try it. If you enjoy it, then stick with it.

In addition, most people feel calm and have a sense of well-being after they exercise. You can actually walk off your anxieties. People who exercise feel better about themselves, look better, feel more energetic, and are more productive at work.

Dr. Colbert Approved

Tips for Sticking With Your Routine

- Don't look at exercise as something you can do in your spare time. Make this time an important part of your day.

- In addition, don't think about it as work. See it as a special time to be alone with God, surrounded by the wonders of His creation. As you exercise, thank God for all of His love for you and for His blessings in your life.

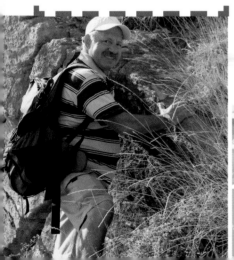

NOW, TAKE THE OFFENSIVE!

TAKE THE OFFENSIVE, AND follow the positive steps suggested in this book. You will discover how effective God's wisdom can be in both the spiritual and natural realms. God heals in many ways, whether through supernatural means or through the more gradual— but equally divine—means of proper nutrition, exercise, and biblical life choices.

Dr. Colbert Approved

Lifestyle Family Fitness Centers

I have worked out at many different gyms and health clubs over the past thirty years, but none have impressed me as much as Lifestyle Family Fitness centers. They have the finest facilities, the best certified personal trainers, and friendly staff and management. Kyle and I highly recommend their centers for those individuals who are ready for intermediate or advanced workouts. Located nationwide, Lifestyle Family Fitness centers are great for the entire family. Visit their Web site at www.lff.com to find a center near you, or call (866) 533-2222.

APPENDIX A

Exercise Contract

I, _____ [print your name], hereby
commit to get fit and live. I understand that according to 1 Corinthians 6:19–20 my body is
not my own, but it was bought by the blood of Jesus. I am to glorify God in my body and
my spirit. With that understanding, I affirm that:

- I commit to reading the entire book *Get Fit and Live!* and practicing the principles that it contains.

- I commit to a regular activity schedule of walking or performing some other aerobic activity for twenty to thirty minutes at least five days a week.

- I commit to performing calisthenics or lifting weights three days a week.

- I commit to following the stretching exercises as outlined in chapter 10 every other day.

- I commit to maintaining a daily exercise/activity diary.

- I commit to visualizing myself at my ideal weight.

- My family is committed to my exercise and activity goals.

- I commit to having an accountability partner.

I understand that failure to comply may sabotage my exercise and workout goals. I
agree to adhere to the above commitments in order to get fit and live.

YOUR SIGNATURE: _____ **DATE:** _____

WITNESS'S SIGNATURE: _____

APPENDIX B

BODY MASS INDEX FOR ADULTS TABLE

BMI Categories

- Underweight = < 18.5
- Normal weight = 18.5–24.9
- Overweight = 25–29.9
- Obesity = BMI of 30 or greater

BMI	Normal						Overweight					Obese									
	19	20	21	22	23	24	25	26	27	28	29	30	31	32	33	34	35	36	37	38	39
Height (inches)									Body Weight (pounds)												
58	91	96	100	105	110	115	119	124	129	134	138	143	148	153	158	162	167	172	177	181	186
59	94	99	104	109	114	119	124	128	133	138	143	148	153	158	163	168	173	178	183	188	193
60	97	102	107	112	118	123	128	133	138	143	148	153	158	163	168	174	179	184	189	194	199
61	100	106	111	116	122	127	132	137	143	148	153	158	164	169	174	180	185	190	195	201	206
62	104	109	115	120	126	131	136	142	147	153	158	164	169	175	180	186	191	196	202	207	213
63	107	113	118	124	130	135	141	146	152	158	163	169	175	180	186	191	197	203	208	214	220
64	110	116	122	128	134	140	145	151	157	163	169	174	180	186	192	197	204	209	215	221	227
65	114	120	126	132	138	144	150	156	162	168	174	180	186	192	198	204	210	216	222	228	234
66	118	124	130	136	142	148	155	161	167	173	179	186	192	198	204	210	216	223	229	235	241
67	121	127	134	140	146	153	159	166	172	178	185	191	198	204	211	217	223	230	236	242	249
68	125	131	138	144	151	158	164	171	177	184	190	197	203	210	216	223	230	236	243	249	256
69	128	135	142	149	155	162	169	176	182	189	196	203	209	216	223	230	236	243	250	257	263
70	132	139	146	153	160	167	174	181	188	195	202	209	216	222	229	236	243	250	257	264	271
71	136	143	150	157	165	172	179	186	193	200	208	215	222	229	236	243	250	257	265	272	279
72	140	147	154	162	169	177	184	191	199	206	213	221	228	235	242	250	258	265	272	279	287
73	144	151	159	166	174	182	189	197	204	212	219	227	235	242	250	257	265	272	280	288	295
74	148	155	163	171	179	186	194	202	210	218	225	233	241	249	256	264	272	280	287	295	303
75	152	160	168	176	184	192	200	208	216	224	232	240	248	256	264	272	279	287	295	303	311
76	156	164	172	180	189	197	205	213	221	230	238	246	254	263	271	279	287	295	304	312	320

BMI	Extreme Obesity														
	40	41	42	43	44	45	46	47	48	49	50	51	52	53	54
Height (inches)							Body Weight (pounds)								
58	191	196	201	205	210	215	220	224	229	234	239	244	248	253	258
59	198	203	208	212	217	222	227	232	237	242	247	252	257	262	267
60	204	209	215	220	225	230	235	240	245	250	255	261	266	271	276
61	211	217	222	227	232	238	243	248	254	259	264	269	275	280	285
62	218	224	229	235	240	246	251	256	262	267	273	278	284	289	295
63	225	231	237	242	248	254	259	265	270	278	282	287	293	299	304
64	232	238	244	250	256	262	267	273	279	285	291	296	302	308	314
65	240	246	252	258	264	270	276	282	288	294	300	306	312	318	324
66	247	253	260	266	272	278	284	291	297	303	309	315	322	328	334
67	255	261	268	274	280	287	293	299	306	312	319	325	331	338	344
68	262	269	276	282	289	295	302	308	315	322	328	335	341	348	354
69	270	277	284	291	297	304	311	318	324	331	338	345	354	358	365
70	278	285	292	299	306	313	320	327	334	341	348	355	362	369	376
71	286	293	301	308	315	322	329	338	343	351	358	365	372	379	386
72	294	302	309	316	324	331	338	346	353	361	368	375	383	390	397
73	302	310	318	325	333	340	348	355	363	371	378	386	393	401	408
74	311	319	326	334	342	350	358	365	373	381	389	396	404	412	420
75	319	327	335	343	351	359	367	375	383	391	399	407	415	423	431
76	328	336	344	353	361	369	377	385	394	402	410	418	426	435	443

APPENDIX C

Recommended Products and Resources

These are products mentioned throughout this book that are also offered through Divine Health.

Divine Health Products
1908 Boothe Circle
Longwood, FL 32750
Phone: (407) 331-7007
Web site: www.drcolbert.com
E-mail: info@drcolbert.com

- **Snack Bars:** Divine Health Snack Bar (chocolate), Divine Health Meal Replacement Bar (peanut butter), Divine Health Enhanced Whey Protein (chocolate or vanilla)

- **Natural Energy Boosters:** Corvalen, Living B_{12}, and Green Tea Elite

- **Pedometer:** Divine Health Pedometer

Additional Products

- **The Seven Pillars of Health Exercise DVD:** Available as a free download from www.sevenpillarsofhealth.com.

- **Exercise Equipment You'll Need for the Get Fit and Live Workout:** A rebounder, stabilizer ball, resistance bands, dumbbells, bosu (intermediate and advanced ONLY), Perfect Pushups (optional, intermediate and advanced ONLY), and an exercise mat (optional).

- **Household Items You'll Need for the Get Fit and Live Workout:** A sturdy chair, phone book (optional), sturdy ottoman or bench, door, and blank wall.

NOTES

Chapter 1
Let's Stir the Waters

1. Don Colbert, *What Would Jesus Eat?* (Nahsville, TN: Thomas Nelson, 2002), 168.

2. Ibid., 168–169.

Chapter 2
The Perks of Regular Exercise

1. PreventDisease.com, "More Evidence That Exercise Prevents Cancer," July 2004, http://preventdisease.com/home/tips42.shtml (accessed August 18, 2006).

2. International Agency for Research on Cancer, *IABC Handbooks of Cancer Prevention, Volume 6: Weight Control and Physical Activity* (Lyon, France: IABC Press, 2001).

3. National Cancer Institute, "Cancer Trends Progress Report—2005 Update," http://progressreport.cancer.gov (accessed January 29, 2006).

4. Anne McTiernan et al., "Recreational Physical Activity and the Risk of Breast Cancer in Postmenopausal Women," *Journal of the American Medical Association* 290, no. 10 (September 10, 2003): 1331–1336.

5. Centers for Disease Control and Prevention, "The Burden of Chronic Diseases as Causes of Death, United States," National and State Perspectives, 2004, http://www.cdc.gov/NCCDPHP/burdenbook2004/Section01/tables.htm

(accessed December 24, 2009).

6. Christiaan Leeuwenburgh et al., "Oxidized Amino Acids in the Urine of Aging Rats: Potential Markers for Assessing Oxidative Stress in Vivo," *American Journal of Physiology: Regulatory, Integrative and Comparative Physiology* 276, no. 1 (January 1999): R128–R135. Viewed online at http://ajpregu.physiology.org/cgi/content/abstract/276/1/R128 (accessed December 24, 2009).

7. Barbara Levine, "Hydration 101: The Case for Drinking Enough Water," http://www.myhealthpointe.com/health_Nutrition_news/index.cfm?Health=10 (accessed December 24, 2009).

8. *Harvard University Gazette*, "It's Never Too Late: Joslin Study Shows Diabetes Sufferers See Major Benefits From Minor Exercise, Weight Loss," December 11, 2003, http://www.news.harvard.edu/gazette/2003/12.11/25-diabetes.html (accessed February 8, 2006).

9. Leeuwenburgh et al., "Oxidized Amino Acids in the Urine of Aging Rats."

10. Christine Brownlee, "Buff and Brainy: Exercising the Body Can Benefit the Mind," *Science News Online* 169, no. 8, (February 25, 2006): http://www.sciencenews.org/ articles/20060225/bob10.asp (accessed July 24, 2006).

11. Tom Lloyd, study published in *The Journal of Pediatrics*, as referenced

in Jeanie Lerche Davis, "Got Exercise? Workouts Better for Bone Health," WebMD, June 11, 2004, http://www.webmd.com/content/Article/88/100005.htm (accessed July 21, 2006).

12. Aetna InteliHealth, "Exercise, Diseases, and Conditions: Digestive," Aetna InteliHealth, http://www.intelihealth.com/IH/ihtIH/WSIHW000/8270/8759/189154.html?d=dmtContent (accessed February 8, 2006).

13. Robert Preidt, "Exercise Eases Digestion Problems in the Obese," American Gastroenterological Association, news release, Oct. 3, 2005, as quoted in HealingWell.com, http://news.healingwell.com/index.php?p=news1&id=528275 (accessed December 28, 2009).

14. S. S. Tworoger et al., "Effects of a Yearlong Moderate-Intensity Exercise and a Stretching Intervention on Sleep Quality in Postmenopausal Women," *Sleep* 26, no. 7 (November 2003): 830–836.

15. Ibid.

16. Associated Press, "Working Out May Help Prevent Colds, Flu: Moderate Exercise Can Boost Body's Defenses, but Too Much Can Be Harmful," MSNBC.com, January 17, 2006, http://www.msnbc.msn.com/id/10894093/ (accessed July 31, 2006).

17. James Blumenthal et al., "Effects of Exercise Training in Older Patients With Major Depression," *Archives of Internal Medicine* 159, no. 19 (1999): 2349–2356.

18. Free Health Encyclopedia, "Physical Fitness—Benefits of Physical Activity and Exercise on the Body," http://www.faqs.org/health/Healthy-Living-V1/Physical-Fitness.html (accessed October 3, 2006).

19. Mayo Clinic Staff, "Chronic Pain: Exercise Can Bring Relief," MayoClinic.com, August 31, 2005, http://www.riversideonline.com/health_reference/Nervous-System/AR00017.cfm (accessed December 28, 2009).

20. Mayo Clinic Staff, "Aerobic Exercise: What 30 Minutes a Day Can Do for Your Body," MayoClinic.com, March 4, 2005, http://www.mayoclinic.com/health/aerobic-exercise/EP00002 (accessed August 29, 2006).

Chapter 3
Before You Begin

1. U. S. Department of Health and Human Services, "Physical Activity Guidelines for Americans," http://www.health.gov/paguidelines/guidelines/chapter6.aspx (accessed December 28, 2009).

2. Elizabeth Quinn, "Proper Hydration for Exercise—Water or Sports Drinks," About.com, June 29, 2009, http://sportsmedicine.about.com/od/hydrationandfluid/a/ProperHydration.htm?p=1 (accessed December 29, 2009).

Chapter 4
How Much Exercise Do You Need?

1. James A. Levine, N. L. Eberhardt, and M. D. Jensen, "Role of Nonexercise Activity Thermogenesis in Resistance to Fat Gain in Humans," *Science* 283 (January 8, 1999): 212–214.

Chapter 5
What Kind of Exercise Do You Need?

1. U. S. Department of Health and Human Services and the U. S. Department of Agriculture, "Dietary Guidelines for Americans 2005: Chapter

4, Physical Activity," http://www.health.gov/dietaryguidelines/dga2005/document/html/chapter4.htm (accessed January 5, 2010).

2. Ralph S. Paffenberger et al., "The Association of Changes in Physical-Activity Level and Other Lifestyle Characteristics With Mortality Among Men," *New England Journal of Medicine* 328, no. 8 (February 1993): 538–545.

3. Jackie Berning, "Strategies for Weight Loss," University of Michigan Health System, http://www.med.umich.edu/1libr/sma/sma_weight_sma.htm (accessed January 5, 2010).

4. Wikipedia, s.v. "Weight Training," http://en.wikipedia.org/wiki/Weight_training (accessed February 17, 2006).

Chapter 6
Fun, Alternative Fitness

1. SahajaYoga.org, "Medical Research on Effects of Sahaja Yoga on Hypertension," Stress Management, http://www.sahajayoga.org.in/StressMgmt.asp (accessed January 5, 2010).

2. Marian S. Garfinke et al., "Yoga-Based Intervention for Carpal Tunnel Syndrome," *Journal of the American Medical Association* 280 (November 11, 1998): 1601–1603.

3. P. Jin, "Changes in Heart Rate, Noradrenaline, Cortisol and Mood During Tai Chi," *Journal of Psychosomatic Research* 33, no. 2 (1989): 197–206.

4. Judith Horstman, "Tai Chi," *Arthritis Today,* http://www.arthritis.org/resources/arthritistoday/2000_archives/2000_07_08_taichi.asp (accessed February 14, 2005). Jacqueline Stenson, "Tai Chi Improves Lung Function in Older

People," *Medical Tribune News Service* (1995). D. D. Brown et al., "Cardiovascular and Ventilatory Responses During Formalized Tai Chi Chuan Exercise," *Research Quarterly for Exercise and Sport* 60, vol. 3 (1989): 246–250.

5. The Pilates Center, "A History of Joseph Hubertus Pilates," http://www.thepilatescenter.com/jhpilates.htm (accessed February 17, 2006).

6. Wikipedia, s.v. "Pilates," http://en.wikipedia.org/wiki/Pilates (accessed February 7, 2006).

7. Charlene Laino, "Wii Games Burn Calories Like a Brisk Walk," WebMD.com, http://www.webmd.com/fitness-exercise/news/20091117/wii-games-burn-calories-like-a-brisk-walk (accessed January 5, 2010).

Chapter 7
The Importance of Correct Posture

1. Thomas Edison, "Laura Moncur's Motivational Quotes," The Quotations Page, http://www.quotationspage.com/quote/38576.html (accessed February 9, 2010).

Chapter 11
Targeting Weight Loss

1. Peter Jaret, "A Healthy Mix of Rest and Motion," *New York Times*, May 3, 2007, http://www.nytimes.com/2007/05/03/fashion/03Fitness.html?adxnnl=1253561931-OZY42iiNSU3WgNPEf4OoxA (accessed September 21, 2009).

Chapter 12
Targeting Type 2 Diabetes

1. Chris Woolston, "Ills and Conditions: Preventing Diabetes Through Diet and Exercise," CVS Pharmacy Health Resources, http://www.cvshealthresources.com/topic/exdiabetes (accessed January 12, 2010).

2. Yuzo Sato, Masaru Nagasaki, Naoya Nakai, and Takashi Fushimi, "Physical Exercise Improves Glucose Metabolism in Lifestyle-Related Diseases," *Experimental Biology and Medicine* 228 (2003): 1208–1212. Available online at http://www.ebmonline.org/cgi/content/abstract/228/10/1208 (accessed January 12, 2010).

3. Ming Wei, Larry W. Gibbons, Tedd L. Mitchell, James B. Kampert, Chong D. Lee, and Steven N. Blair, "The Association Between Cardiorespiratory Fitness and Impaired Fasting Glucose and Type 2 Diabetes Mellitus in Men," *Annals of Internal Medicine* 130, no. 2 (January 19, 1999): 89–96. Available online at http://www.ncbi.nlm.nih.gov/pubmed/10068380 (accessed July 29, 2009).

4. Berit L. Heitmann and Peder Fredericksen, "Thigh Circumference and Risk of Heart Disease and Premature Death: Prospective Cohort Study," *BMJ* 339 (September 3, 2009). Available online at http://www.bmj.com/cgi/content/abstract/339/sep03_2/b3292 (accessed September 21, 2009).

5. L. E. Davidson, R. Hudson, K. Kilpatrick, et al., "Effects of Exercise Modality on Insulin Resistance and Functional Limitation in Older Adults: A Randomized Controlled Trial," *Archives of Internal Medicine* 169, no. 2 (2009): 122–131. Available online at http://archinte.ama-assn.org/cgi/content/abstract/169/2/122 (accessed July 31, 2009).

Chapter 13
Targeting Osteoporosis

1. Melinda Thompson, "Weight Bearing Exercises," Suite101.com, http://womenshealth.suite101.com/article.cfm/weight_bearing_exercises (accessed July 6, 2009).

Chapter 15
Targeting Heart Disease

1. "High Blood Pressure Overview," NYTimes.com, http://health.nytimes.com/health/guides/disease/hypertension/lifestyle-changes.html?print=1 (accessed January 13, 2010).

2. Judy Ismach, "No Two Genders About It, a Heart Is Just a Heart," *Physician's Weekly* 14, no. 10 (February 10, 1997). Available online at http://www.physweekly.com/archive/97/02_10_97/itn1.html (accessed February 16, 2006).

Chapter 16
Targeting Cancer

1. "Physical Activity and the Cancer Patient," American Cancer Society, http://www.cancer.org/docroot/mit/content/mit_2_3x_physical_activity_and_the_cancer_patient.asp (accessed January 13, 2010).

2. Ibid.

3. Ibid.

4. "Bounce Back Into Shape" *Prevention* magazine 52, no. 52 (March 2000): 91.

Conclusion

1. MU News Bureau, "Daily Dog Walks Work Off Weight for Owners, MU Researchers Find," University of Missouri—Columbia, Sinclair School of Nursing, September 28, 2005, http://www.cvm.missouri.edu/News/dailydogwalks.htm (accessed January 13, 2010).

2. Elizabeth Quinn, "Delayed Onset Muscle Soreness: Dealing With Muscle Pain After Exercise," About: Sports Medicine, http://sportsmedicine.about.com/cs/injuries/a/aa010600.htm (accessed February 17, 2006).

A Personal Note

From Don Colbert

YOU MAY HAVE NOTICED at the beginning of this book that I've dedicated it to my father, Don Colbert Sr. From the moment my father gave his heart to Jesus he was a radiant witness for Christ. I used to get so embarrassed as a teenager because my father would witness to complete strangers every day. Even more embarrassing was when he witnessed to my friends! He would ask them, "Have you made your reservation?"

They would look at him, puzzled, and reply, "To what?" I knew they were trying to remember if there was a new concert in town.

My father would smile at them and say, "Your reservation to the marriage supper of the Lamb." Then he would share Jesus with them. Many accepted his invitation, both strangers and friends alike.

Now, like my dad, I ask you, "Have *you* made *your* reservation?"

If you haven't met my best friend, Jesus, I would like to take this opportunity to introduce Him to you. It is very simple. If you are ready to let Him come into your life and become your best friend, all you need to do is sincerely pray this prayer:

> *Lord Jesus, I want to know You as my Savior and Lord. I believe You are the Son of God and that You died for my sins. I also believe You were raised from the dead and now sit at the right hand of the Father praying for me. I ask You to forgive me for my sins and change my heart so that I can be Your child and live with You eternally. Thank You for Your peace. Help me to walk with You so that I can begin to know You as my best friend and my Lord. Amen.*

If you have prayed this prayer, you have just made the most important decision of your life. I rejoice with you in your decision and your new relationship with Jesus. Please contact my publisher at pray4me@strang.com so that we can send you some materials that will help you become established in your relationship with the Lord. We look forward to hearing from you.

Simple,
delicious,
healthy food choices
from the author of
The Seven Pillars of Health

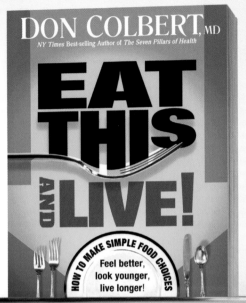

New York Times best-selling author Dr. Don Colbert gives you the information you need to make healthy food choices every day. *Eat This and Live!* teaches you what the Bible has to say about food and gives Dr. Colbert's recommendations on which foods to eat heartily, eat in moderation, or avoid.

Visit your local bookstore to get the tools **YOU NEED** for healthier living.

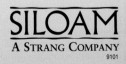

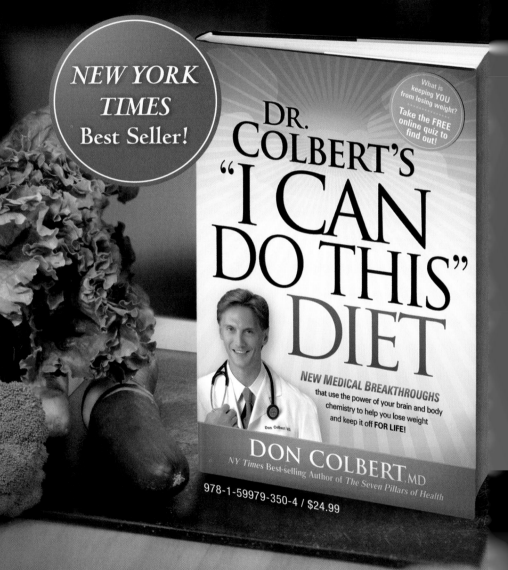

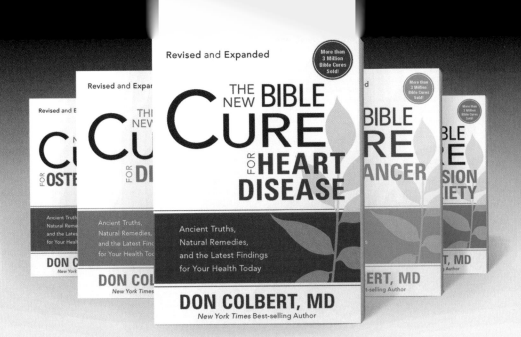

YOU WANT TO BE HEALTHY. GOD WANTS YOU TO BE HEALTHY.

In each book of the Bible Cure series, you will find helpful alternative medical information together with uplifting and faith-building biblical truths.

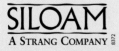